buRNoUT

buRNoUT

TIME TO MAKE A YOU TURN

Danny Demeersseman

PROGRAM BOOKET

PRESENTATION
OF THE EXHIBITION

BECOME ACQUAINTED
WITH YOUR GUIDE

Danny Demeersseman (1964) has a practice as psychologist and certified massage therapist in Belgium where he combines coaching with therapeutic massage.

He likes to walk with people through their inner wilderness and teach them how to discover peace and create structure in life. The writer in Danny finds it challenging to travel to unknown worlds and then enthusiastically guidehis readers around.

He has published several books on massage, education, psychology and poetry.

In this book he navigates you through the imaginary exhibition 'Burnout: time to make a you turn". Together with his alter ego Don Key you'll make a unique journey to your inner self, to the caterpillar in you. This way you'll discover how buRNoUT challenges you to TURN yourself into a unique butterfly.

"The highest happiness of man
is to be found only in his personality."
- Johann Wolfgang von Goethe -

This work was born after intense showers of thinking, feeling, daring, doing and, above all, starting over and over again. There were gusts of enthusiasm, frustration, self-pity, joy, satisfaction, doubt, pride, shyness, surprise,…in short the fickleness of life.

DANNY DEMEERSSEMAN ON AMAZON

I've developed several fields of interest: massage, healing, health, education, poetry...

You may find an overview of my eBooks on http://www.amazon.com/-/e/B00MUPAR2O:

My eBooks on massage:

- 50 Techniques for Shiatsu Chair Massage
- Abdominal Massage Course
- Integrated Head Massage

My eBooks on education:

- Math Number Houses
- Parent Guide for Multiplication Tables

My eBooks on psychology:

- How to Beat Procrastination?
- The Stress Management Suitcase

My eBooks on poetry:

- 120 Modern Christmas Wishes for Greeting Cards:
- 90 Wishes for Happy New Year Greeting Cards
- 210 Christmas and New Year Wishes for Greeting Cards
- 120 Condolence Poems for Sympathy Cards
- More than 300 Wishes for Birthday Greetings

WORDS OF GRATITUDE

In particular, I appreciate the support of my girlfriend Priscilla, who regularly held my head above the water while writing this life-swimming course. I thank my clients for the authenticity and sincerity of their life stories.

Due to the fresh look of several test readers spelling errors were corrected and the structure of the book received a complete face-lift.

My sincere thanks to you all.

"When the sun doesn't shine,
then dance in the rain."
- Don Key -

Danny Demeersseman
www.learnandenjoy.com

DISCOVER THE GROUNDS OF THIS EXHIBITION

Before Don Key, your guide, gives you a tour through the exhibition 'Burnout: time to make a turn', we like to present the vision of our museum for health and well-being. Then you'll be better informed to decide if you really want to visit our expo around burn out!

OUR METHOD

Do not expect an exhibition in the form of an all-inclusive holiday where vitality is served on your bed as breakfast.

Do you wish to embark on a cruise with eternal energy as your final destination, then you have booked the wrong trip. We apologize for your inconvenience.

Do you expect short travel trips, which will require little effort and provide you with a 100% satisfaction money-back guarantee, thenwe can't help you. Sorry again!

What can you expect from us? Our journey will invite you to reconnect with yourself. Sometimes you'll be rowing with headwind, occasionally you'll need to row back, now and again you'll have to anchor, ... but there will also be sufficient time for sunbathing on the deck, enjoying the views or meeting nice people.

So you'll discover that you need to make a u (you) turn in your life. After all, the letters of the word 'turn' are hidden in the term 'buRNoUT'. This journey will lead you back to your inner self, if you really dare to unfold yourself and give meaning to your life and to that of others in an authentic way. So you must resolutely walk the path of self-realization.

This book will give you new shoes. So your current running style will be transformed into a walking style that suits you. Your life path will change into a beautiful, wide avenue with convenient side streets and inviting resting benches.

The doubts you're feeling now are completely normal and are part of change process in life. So there is absolutely no reason to panic! Don Key, your guide, has tons of experience to expertly guide you through the burn out swamp. His uplifting motto is after all:

> *"If you find shit on your path,*
> *then use it as manure."*
> **- JaapBressers-**

By visiting this exhibition, you unravel the message of burnout and, on your path to self-realization, you become acquainted with important allies like mindfulness, dosage, gratitude, self-love, acceptance, authenticity, compassion, vulnerability, courage, connecting, commitment, ...

A SHORT OVERVIEW OF THE EXHIBITION

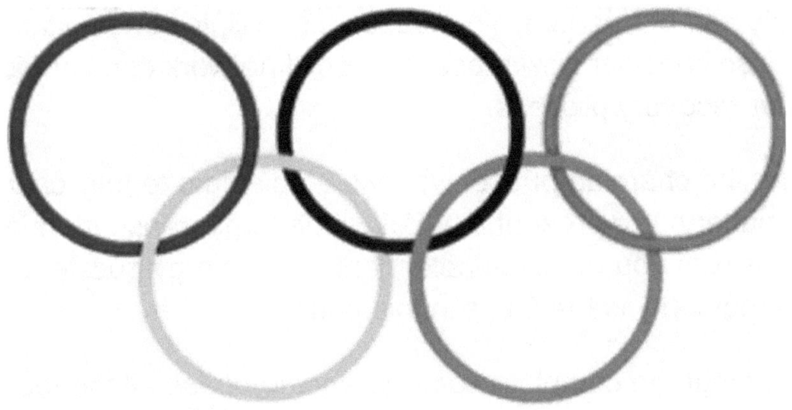

At the entrance of the exhibition you recognize the logo of the Olympic Games. We use this symbol to indicate that you will not automatically recover from a burnout. You must patiently and conscientiously follow an adjusted training schedule. Preferably under the guidance of a professional coach.

The five rings represent the five phases that form the framework of our burnout approach. We distinguish 5 c's: the Contemplation phase, the Charging phase, the Comprehending phase, the Commitment phase and finally the Consolidating phase.

In the *contemplation phase* we reply to the question "*What does a burnout want to tell you?*" We also focus on the acceptance process of this radical wake-up call.

Once you recognize and accept that burnout is a safety system of your body to prevent further disaster, you will realize that your life is in need of a thorough restyling and that external help is indispensable.Therefore, take an experienced coach to help you

coordinate your personality, work and personal situation.
Together with you, he will look at how a more favorable work life
climate can be created. Your supervisor will, in consultation with
you, also consider how a positive social network can contribute
to your recovery process.

During the charging phase, we take ample time to fully charge
your battery. We present a buffet with energy transmitters and
discuss with you the avoidable menu with energy guzzlers.
Daily regularity is the focus in this phase.

Throughout the complete *comprehending phase* all the facets
that are related to burnout are fully explored. We place your
brain under a microscope and look for beliefs that you
sometimes apply too stubbornly, so they obstruct your life, like
the conviction "*Everything has to go perfectly*" or the opinion
"*Others must always like me.*"

In this phase you have to make crucial decisions to tackle
burnout by replacing these negative beliefs with realistic,
positive statements such as "Efficiency is important, but
perfection is unrealistic" or "It's nice that some people like me
and it's normal that not everyone likes me."

In the *commitment phase* you gradually start working again.
Thanks to new building materials such as acceptance, self-love,
forgiveness, dosage, compassion, gratitude, authenticity,
courage, self-realization, ... your immune system regains its
much needed fuel, your nervous system retrieves its balance
and your stress level drops. Gradually, enthusiasm is bubbling
into your blood vessels again.

Parallel to this commitment phase starts the consolidating phase, in which you closely monitor how your new ME is capable of keeping negative stress within acceptable limits, walking often enough on quiet paths and taking up achievable challenges.

Realize that relapse is very real, but not disastrous! Be patient and not overconfident! Learn from the past and from the now. Discover which keys give access to real happiness. "*Try to be a donkey,*" says Don Key smiling "*and do not knock twice against the burnout stone.*"

HOW DO YOU GET THE BIGGEST BENEFIT FROM OUR EXHIBTION?

We advise you to take sufficient time between the different chapters. It is even worthwhile to re-read some parts. This way you can test how far you have already succeeded in integrating certain new ideas into your life.

As mentioned above, you get more out of this book if you let yourself be guided by a therapist. A coach can help you clarify certain matters and encourage you as a supporter during your life triathlon, which consists of the disciplines *'Deliberate your options, Value your feelingsand Do different things'*. That way the DVD of your new life becomes a real blockbuster!

Finally, unlike taking medicines, you can advise everyone to visit this exhibition, even several times. There is no danger of overdose. Afterwards it can be enriching to exchange experiences among each other.

People who do not have a burnout may also benefit from this exhibition. They will (re) discover the booby traps of our modern society and learn how they can better protect themselves against pitfalls.

CONTEMPLATION PHASE

SEEK PROFESSIONAL HELP

Enteringthe first hall of the exhibition we are treated to applause. Allowing a coach to guide you is not an easy step. It requires courage and deserves congratulations.

Try to see APPlause as a fantastic app to share with others, but definitely download it for yourself and use it daily.

On top of this unexpected acclaim we receive a mirror as a gift. It is a symbol that represents the intention of therapy.

> *"Professional help is a reflection*
> *of your own Deliberations, Values and Doings*
> *with the freedom to direct*
> *your own life movie."*
> **- Don Key -**

Maybe it is difficult for you to accept support. Someone who is naturally inclined to offer help sometimes finds it difficult to receive and request assistance. The false beliefs mentioned below often stop us from being open to assistance.

- I do not want to be dependent on others.
- I tend to solve everything myself and that usually works well.
- My problem is not severe enough to ask for help.
- My situation is too specific to be understood by others.

Do you recognize these limiting ideas when you look at yourself? Then drop them and search for positive thoughts, as listed below, which lower the threshold to accept support:

- *Getting help* means that a co-driver is sitting next to me. The wheel of my life remains in my own hands.
- Everyone asks for assistance, especially in difficult situations. For example, there is no top athlete who says: "*I do not need a coach!*"
- I leave the responsibility to the care provider to indicate which assistance he can or can't provide.
- A coach can broaden my view. The worst problems do not usually resolve themselves by searching for answers, but by getting started with new, never-asked questions.
- With a request for support, I give myself the following message: "*I deserve to be happier.*"
- *Asking for help*requires courage. This is a quality that I can be proud of!

Enabling professional support is like booking a trip with a guide. You discover a lot more, no unnecessary time is lost, your attention is focused on interesting things that would otherwise not stand out, you can always ask for clarification, ...

2

FIND THE MISSION OF BURNOUT

Leaving the room about professional help we end up in a narrow corridor. As soon as we enter it, the light dims. Youanxiouslygrabmy hand and we suddenly stop. It seems that this helps. As soon as we do not move or step carefully, it stops getting darker in the corridor. Halfway down thehallway we see a button with the label *extra energy*. And yes, indeed! With the press of that button the original light intensity is restored. Our joy is only short-lived. When we continue walking now, it becomes even darker than before. Just before it is completely dark, we are relieved to reach the end of the corridor. There we find a sign with the slogan:

> *"Watch out! Borrowing energy also costs energy!"*
> **- Don Key -**

This was a confrontational experience for both of us. The solution method *switching to a higher gear*has its limits. Continuouslyaddressingyour energy reserves does notremain unpunished.

Why is it that, against better judgment, we often continue to choose an approach that yields no results? Why is it so difficult for many to say stop or no and change course?

Making decisions we mainly count on our internal library with *personal beliefs*. These *claims*, which we have built up over the years, have a strong truth-character. We almost follow them blindly to make decisions and take actions in our lives.

In the lessons above you have experienced that the belief "*if something does not work, switch to a higher gear*" can be a negative opinion that can set you back in achieving your goals.

If you want to reduce negative stress, you have to dig deep into yourself to bring this belief system to the surface, in order to reveal the message of your burnout. Ask yourself the following question: "*Which of my statements are so convincing that they keep my life under control and prevent me from taking other directions?*"

The willingness to question these personal ideas and, where necessary, to adjust them, often proves to be a necessary step to normalize stress and to reduce or prevent burnout.

> *"A 'No' uttered from the deepest conviction*
> *is better than a 'Yes' merely uttered to please,*
> *or worse, to avoid trouble!"*
> **- Mahatma Gandhi -**

In the remainder of this exhibition, we will regularly reflect on this powerful belief system.

TRY TO UNDERSTAND STRESS BURNOUT

Entering the next room we receive a sealed pair of glasses. We are instructed to step on a treadmill and reach the other side of the hall as quickly as possible. We can not see through the glasses and we only have a beeping signal as an aid.

We begin this task with great enthusiasm, but our joy is short-lived when we realize that the treadmill suddenly changes direction. The harder we run, the faster the treadmill reverts, so that we remain on the same spot. We even lose ground due to fatigue, something that this idiotic treadmill does not know.

"*Aha,*" you suddenly shout, "*this is a déjàvu experience.*" You think of the narrow corridor of the previous room, where it got darker as you stepped. We then learned that our energy tank is not a bottomless vessel.

When we have just caught our breath, you notice that you can peek past the sides of your glasses. You discover that the treadmill has a wide edge on both sides and you propose to reach the other side by stepping on the two edges next to the treadmill. Now the reverse direction of the treadmill can no longer hinder us in reaching the other side of the room.

With the necessary laughter, but as two proud peacocks, we reach the other side of the hall. This thanks to your courage to think out of the box.

*"Our head is round so our thoughts
can change direction!"*
- Rainer Maria Rilke -

Thinking differently is the most important medicine to avoid or to combat burnout. If you continue to cling to familiar thinking routes as an autopilot and are not willing to take over the control stick sometimes, when you have new insights, then burnout will force you into an emergency landing.

Now we continue with discussinghow stress and burnout develop using a simple scheme: Albert Ellis's ABC model of stress and burnout.

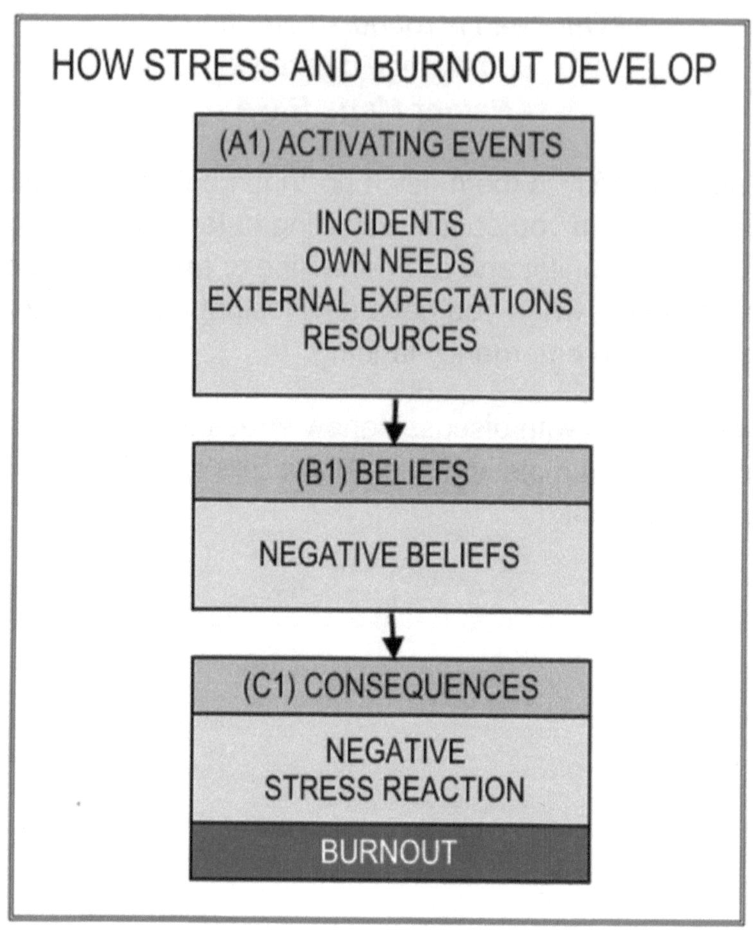

ACTIVATING EVENTS

Activating events are neutral elements on which you will pass judgment. These subjective judgments, called beliefs, ultimately determine which form of stress (= positive or negative) you will experience.

In a situation we can distinguish four types of activating: incidents, own needs, external expectations and internal / external resources.

We give an example of the four types of activating events

- *Incidents*: for example, there is more work due to a colleague's illness.
- *Own needs*: for example, you have a great need for self-development.
- *External expectations*: for example, you have to pick up the children quickly after work, because your partner has no time.
- *Resources*:for example, you can count on support and understanding from your partner (= external resource) or you know that you are handy in determining priorities (= internal resource).

There is also an interaction between the four activating events. Ask yourself regularly "*To what extent do I think incidents, external expectations and internal / external resources make it possible to fulfill my own needs?*"

BELIEFS THAT ARE NEGATIVE

Activating events are provided by you with a negative or a positive belief according to whether they favor or not fulfill your own needs.

We will repeat the examples and provide them with a possible negative or possible positive belief.

ACTIVATING EVENT	NEGATIVE BELIEF	POSITVE BELIEF
Incident: there is more work due to a colleague's illness,	I'm so busy and now this. It is too much.	A unique challenge to prove myself.
Own need: I have a great need for self-development.	There are never opportunities to do my own thing.	I will find a way to do my own thing.
External expectation: my partner wants me to pick up the children.	I always have to solve everything. I can not handle it.	If I only do the important work, I will succeed.
External resource: I can count on the help of my partner.	That support means that I can not handle it myself. How bad!	The help of people proves that they like me.
Internal resource: I can determine what is important.	Because of this quality, everyone wants to benefit from me.	Because of this quality, I can handle the extra work.

Here again you can clearly see that incidents, own needs, external expectations and external or internal resources, through a different interpretation, can give rise to beliefs that vary from person to person and that in terms of content can be prohibitive or helpful.

> *"It is very rare or almostimpossible*
> *that an **event** can be negative*
> *from all points of view."*
> **- Dalai Lama -**

We end here with a brief overview of common annoying and supportive beliefs.

Examples of annoying, negativebeliefs

- I'mnotgoodenough.
- Nobodylikes me.
- Everything must be perfect.
- Success is not for me.
- I am afraid of change.
- Conflictsscare me off.

Examples of supportive, *positive beliefs*

- I can change.
- I am worthy to love.
- I trust myself.
- I respect myself as I am.
- I dare to give affection.
- The future can still go in all directions.

You will meanwhile have understood that negative beliefs trigger a negative stress reaction that can lead to burnout and that positive beliefs try to avoid this.

CONSEQUENCES THAT ARE NEGATIVE

Your belief system has important consequences. If you interpret Activating events (A), then, according to your interpretation, negative or positive Beliefs (B) arise, which as a Consequence (C) cause a negative or positive stress response.

So activating events never are the cause of your stress, but for sure your beliefs, your interpretations of these events are the cause. This is an extremely important starting point in our approach to handle stress and burnout.

We distinguish two possible stress reactions.

- A *positive stressreaction*: helping insights provide dosed physical sensations and emotions. These form a favorable breeding ground for constructive behavior and open the way to self-realization.
- A *negative stressreaction*: obstructing beliefs develop unpleasant physical sensations and feelings that can be extreme. These reactions increase the risk of destructive behavior. In the long term this can lead to burnout.

Our personal beliefs determine how we experience reality. They decide whether we experience negative or positive stress, whether that tension is high or low and what actions we will take.

> *"People do not get upset by activating events,*
> *but by the way they look at those events."*
> **- based on Epictetus -**

But what is actually happening in our body during a stress response and what is the purpose of this mechanism?

STRESS

When stress takes control of your life, your nervous system brings your body into a higher state of readiness. Your energy tank is refilled. Blood is withdrawn from your organs and sent to your muscles. Your pupils dilate and your blood pressure and heartbeat increase. The adrenal glands are instructed to produce cortisol, a stress hormone. This substance gives you extra force and strengthens your immune system. You are ready for battle.

A stress response also increases your vigilance and gives you the much needed power to respond appropriately at an appropriate time by fighting, fleeing or freezing. We call this the *'fight flight freeze' response*.

Stress is therefore an auxiliary mechanism, whereby your body adjusts when circumstances ask for it.

But why is it that stress sometimes results in a burnout and can you prevent this in one way or another?

FROM STRESS TO BURNOUT

On first view, stress seems to be a useful system to save us from difficult situations. But where does it go wrong in our modern society?

We are overstimulated every day. Our stress system is becoming more and more sensitive and is making more and more overtime. There is not enough time to recover. For example, if you do not repay a loan, but go to another bank for an additional credit, you create a similar unsustainable situation.

In his quest for extra energy, your body draws from the supply of fuel that is actually intended for your recovery and immune system. This will make you even more vulnerable. It goes from bad to worse. You end up in a state of chronic stress.

Your ability to invent and execute effective actions is decreasing. You will no longer be able to stop the stress train. A crash in the form of a burnout is unavoidable if you do not act drastically!

If stress is too often present, takes too high levels and is insufficiently tackled, your body can not and will not wait any longer. It then grabs the emergency brake by means of a burnout. This is a necessary evil to prevent greater calamity. Even positive stress can overturn you by, for example, seducing you through obsession with extreme passion.

It is understandable that, in a first reaction, you regard burnout as a bogeyman. As someone who does not take into account your unfortunate situation and pays little attention to the efforts you make to turn the tide.

Belief me, burnout is not a bully and certainly not a criminal judge. Try to consider burnout as a worried parent who no longer wants to see how you sink further and further into an endless stress swamp and therefore drastically intervenes out of love so that you would realize that drastic adjustments are needed to feel solid ground under your feet again.

Burnout is an ingenious security system of your stress mechanism. It is a kind of safety valve that comes into effect during radical events, if you place high demands on yourself, in case of workload, in case of insufficient rest, little help, negative beliefs, ...

If you do not correctly interpret formal notices with warning signs such as sleep problems, stomach disorders, fatigue, etc., burnout will act as a debt collector to prevent worse.

Below we show again the ABC model that represents how stress and burnout develop.

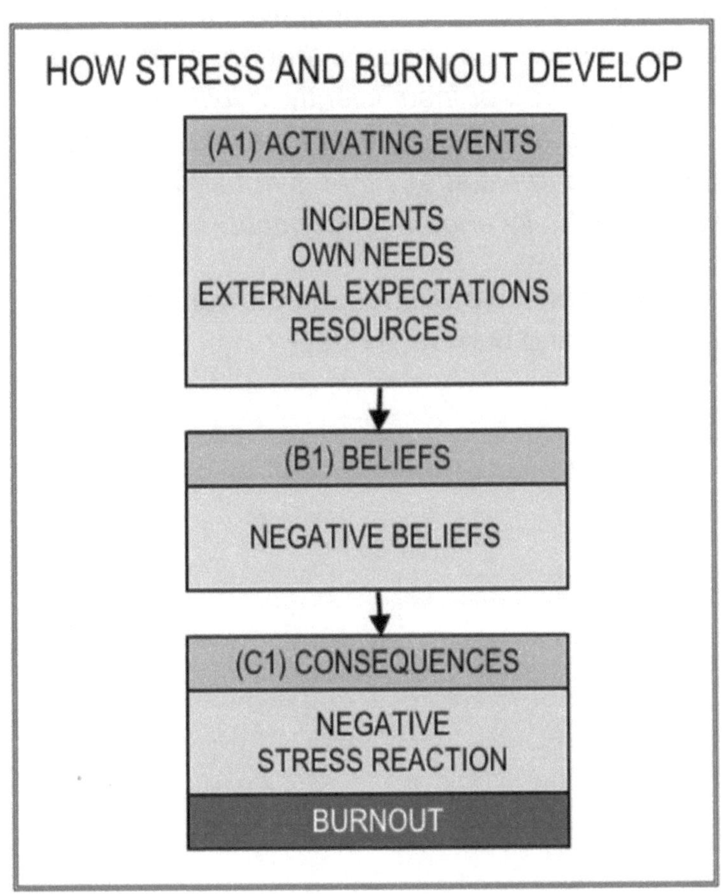

A negative stress reaction proceeds as follows.

- *Activating events* (A) create a field of tension. You ask yourself the question: "*To what extent do incidents, external expectations and resources allow me to set up positive actions to fulfill my own needs?*"
- As a result *negative beliefs* (B) can arise or be triggered. These inhibiting views are so powerful that you trust and act on them blindly.
- *The consequences (C) include negative stress, sensations, emotions and actions that are obstructive. They do not help you or insufficiently in fulfilling your needs and taking external expectations into account. High, negative, chronic stress that is not effectively addressed eventually ends up irrevocably in a burnout.*

In the *comprehending phase* we will deepen the various elements of this stress and burnout model.

ACCEPT YOUR BURNOUT

The goal of the contemplation phase is to give a clear view of your current situation. By understanding how burnout develops, you learn to accept that certain things are currently not achievable and also undesirable.

If your car, computer or mobile phone fails, you try to find out what is going on. You want clarity. First you look at how you can solve this yourself. You may consult the manual. If this fails, you go to the garage or the store where you have bought your car, tablet or phone.

Something similar is happening to you now. You can not manage to turn the tide. The problems do not ebb away spontaneously. Sometimes they become even more abundant and then overwhelm you with violent emotions and disturbing thoughts, which make you powerless.

We have already pointed out that it is high time / high tide for professional support, because a burnout storm is too complex to defy on your own. If this has not happened yet, drop anchor and consult an experienced coach who can sail with you through your questions.

If you experience something serious, then your head turns into a question machine: "*What is happening to me? Why me? How can I solve this as quickly as possible?*" These questions illustrate what you experience, things that currently not seem achievable, the influence of this on others, the uncertain future, ...

During an acceptance process you more or less go through a fixed process: *denying burnout, feeling anger, negotiating, experiencing grief and/or depression and finally accepting burnout.*

The duration and the intensity of each stage vary from person to person. Stages can also overlap.

DENYING

We enter a new room. There is a thick layer of sand on the ground. Suddenly there is a deafening noise through the loudspeakers. We spontaneously put our hands on our ears. We can just suppress the tendency to put our head in the sand.

We have met the first phase that we go through when accepting burnout: *denying*.

During a burnout you go through a coping process. Annie Romein-Verschoor describes it as follows: "*At every difficult crossroads of your life you lose a part of yourself. You no longer have contact with your own identity. You sit at home and your head screams: 'This does not happen to me!'*"

You put your head in the sand and refuse to face reality. Denial is a normal form of self-protection. It helps you, as long as you do not get stuck in it, to decide for yourself at what rate feelings and thoughts are admitted.

Tame the tendency to understand everything directly and completely and tame the tendency to bend the future in a certain direction. Let go of the past and the future and connect with the present!

FEELING ANGER

As soon as the severity of a burnout pervades, anger often comes up with the question "*Why me?*" You can get angry at yourself, your employer, your colleagues, your housemates, ...Feelings of resentment, envy and indignation may arise . You can feel overwhelmed by powerlessness.

There are various ways to express your anger. You can respond passively by ignoring your anger, blaming yourself, giving up or avoiding things. You can also respond actively with revenge, shouting, physical aggression or accusing others of something. This is understandable, but it is more beneficial to express your feelings through writing, talking, crying, light movement, yoga, meditation, ...

Under that envy and frustration are feelings like sadness, fear, pain, ... Try to connect with those feelings. Experience step by step the sadness, the fear or the pain under your anger. These emotions beg for recognition. By feeling you can move the energy of your emotions and you can transform them more easily. The meaning of the word emotion derives from the Latin word *émovéré*, which you can translate as *energy in motion*. Feelings therefore serve to re-activate blocked energy.

If you accept that the world is not always fair and honest, you usually make better choices. You then put things more into perspective by saying to yourself, for example: "I find my boss annoying, but fortunately the job is nice."

Make sure your anger does not turn into a boomerang. Anger contains the danger of self-destruction. It can make you the victim of your own anger.

"Holding onto anger is like drinking poison
and expecting the other person to die."
- Boeddha –

NEGOTIATING

In the third phase of your coping process with burnout you try to control the terrible reality by negotiating. You come up with all kinds of proposals in an attempt to straighten out the situation. You hope tobe able to glue the broken vase.

You promise to do things do change the situation. "What if ... then I am prepared to ..." By creating these what-if proposals, you try to suppress your sense of powerlessness. You are looking for a way out. You want to feel that you're back in control over your life.

By imposing promises on yourself, you create an imaginary reality that is much softer than the harsh reality you are experiencing now. This way of thinking helps you to bridge difficult moments, but lacks a sense of reality to find useful solutions in the long term.

In this phase many people place God or another higher being in the role of mediator. In Him they see their last straw.

EXPERIENCING GRIEF AND/OR DEPRESSION

If you notice that denying, being angry and / or negotiating do not produce results, then often sadness and sometimes depression lurk around the corner.

People with a burnout sometimes mourn about what has happened and can be skeptical about the future. A good social network can provide the necessary support in this phase!

In this stage of coping with burnout you can be overwhelmed by emotions like regret, shame and even fear. Experiences from the past can be retriggered.

The danger exists that you will remain in this phase. It is a matter of staying calm and realizing that you occasionally have to row carefully against the flow of life. Keep going, even if it is difficult and you do not feel like it. Pull yourself out of this vortex by looking for distractions with your family, friends, colleagues, ... Dare to talk about your feelings!

In this phase, people with burnout have a need for a listening ear. If you want to help a person with burnout avoid the helpers' reflex in the sense of softening, predicting a better future or coming up with all kinds of tips.It is better to show understanding and sympathy for the grief.

ACCEPTING

Now you are in the final phase. Allyourfeelings have been put into words. If you have had enough time and help to go through the past stages, you are beginning to gradually accept reality as it is.

You finally feel that you can pick up the thread of your life again. It is a state of surrender to things that you have no control over and a start of believing in new opportunities.

You learn to let things go by giving them a different meaning. This opens the door to a new life.

"Loss is not a loss ifit erases illusions
and shows the way to a better life."
- based on Herbert George Wells -

The five phases of acceptance are rarely followed in a fixed order or with the same intensity and duration. They can also overlap. So there are big individual differences.

Sometimes you think you have accepted a situation and then you are thrown back again to a previous stage. Stabilityrequires time and patience!

CHARGING
PHASE

START AT THE BEGINNING

We take the escalator to the first floor and end up in the *charging phase*, the second phase of the burnout recovery program.

A friendly lady receives us with a big smile in a room that is decorated as a relaxation room. She explains the purpose of the charging phase: "*This phase is a necessary preparation before you start the burnout recovery program. Just as anathlete takes rest and takes good care of himself before he takes part in an important race, so you also have to refuel first before you are able to go deeper into all aspects that are related to the recovery of your burnout.*"

Believe me, you do not win a mountain stage on an empty stomach and to climb out of the valley of a burnout and to avoid relapse in the future, even a full stomach is insufficient. Youalsoneed reserve food.

If your energy level is sufficiently, then it is essential to adopt an attitude in which you carefully monitor your energy level.

INCREASE YOUR ENERGY LEVEL

A car without petrol or a smartphone with empty battery have in common that they no longer work. They both need energy to function again and/or need to be checked whether there is a dysfunction somewhere.

Someone with a burnout finds himself in a similar situation. Considering what is the cause of that burnout, how you can recover and how you can avoid relapse, requires a lot of strength. You currently do not have this energy. So first charging is the only and right decision in the initial phase of overcoming burnout!

Alternate relaxing activities with the focus on enjoyment with short, strenuous activities that are not too intensive. Your energy supply can only recover in this cautious way. Doing nothing all day is certainly not an option. This actually encourages fatigue.

We can call on various energy suppliers. We will discuss the following energy suppliers.

- Learn to enjoy again and experience the benefits of rest and relaxation.
- Alternate this with gradually improving your condition.
- Invest in a good night's sleep.
- Care for healthy food.
- Follow a brain diet.
- Stop multitasking.
- Limit the number of stimuli.

- Live mindful.
- Taste the value of gratitude and discover now-happiness.
- Maintain good social contacts.

Finally, experience the importance of regularity and always keep a close eye on your energy level.

RELEARN TO RELAX AND HAVE FUN

For many people it is difficult to enjoy and say *no* to requests of others and to free up time for themselves. Enjoying also means avoidingmultitasking.

In addition, you must regularly say *no* to your own exaggerated beliefs that put you in second place, like the statement "*I must always be ready for someone else.*"

Below you will find some suggestions to treat yourself and to find the necessary rest and relaxation.

- Pamper yourself with a massage or pay a visit to a sauna center.
- Rediscover nature as an ideal source of energy.
- Choose for quiet sports like walking, cycling or swimming.
- Dance and listen to nice music.
- Surround yourself regularly with positive people.
- Bring humor into your life. Take a look at a comedy or relive funny moments from your life by recalling them.

- Nest yourself in your most lazy armchair with a relaxing book.

You can extend this list with your own ideas.

IMPROVE YOUR CONDITION

Try to gradually improve your body condition by moving or exercising every day. If you are physically recovered, your mental possibilities, for example your concentration, will also increase. Aim for a healthy mind in a healthy body.

Good fitness through movement and sport is a buffer against stress. It is advisable to take half an hour of daily time for short, light physical training through, for example, walking, cycling, swimming or practicing yoga.

Move just enough to sweat and make your heart beat faster. Avoid efforts that make you feel dizzy or short of breath. Regularity is important. First gradually build up the duration of the effort and then gradually increase the intensity. After exercising you need to provide sufficient rest. Learn to alternate between exercise and relaxation.

Walking in nature creates a quiet mood. In addition, you get daylight and you breathe healthy air. Yoga or qi gong provide smooth muscles and reduce stress.

Choose a movement activity that you like. This makes it easier to sustain. Dancing, swimming and gardening are also suitable ways to improve your condition.

If necessary, contact a sports center to conduct an exercise test to determine your level and to draw up an adjusted training schedule.

INVEST IN A GOO NIGHT'S SLEEP

Sleep is a medication that has no side effects and is available without a prescription. Producingthis medicinesometimes requires the necessary exercise and patience. Try these tips below to improve your night's sleep.

- Sleep as much as you like, but follow fixed hours.
- Go to bed earlier than planned if you feel drowsy. Listen toyour body!
- Only keep a siesta when your night's sleep is optimal.
- Provide sufficient physical exercises during the day, but also provide the necessary breaks.
- End your day with relaxation such as a short evening walk, a warm bath or meditation.
- Avoid snacks, television, coffee, smoking, intensive exercises, activities that require a lot of concentration and alcohol one hour before bedtime.
- Avoid, especially in the evening, excessive exposure to the harsh light of television, computer, smartphone, ...
- Provide daylight as soon as you get up to balance your biorhythm. There are alsospecial wake-up lampsforthis.
- Tune your thoughts so you do not worry.
- Choose a light read book to relax your thoughts.
- Sleep in a cool, well-ventilated, quiet and dark room.

- Reserve your bedroom for sleeping and making love. Your partner is an ideal sleeping pill.
- Use a cherry pit pillow if you suffer from cold feet.
- In case of insomnia problems you can apply the following technique.
    - If you do not sleep after 20 minutes, get up and do something relaxing. No TV!
    - If you become drowsy, go back to bed.
    - If you do not sleep again after 20 minutes, repeat this procedure.

  This method works well, but you have to keep it going for two to three weeks.Our body needs time to adjust.
- Consider a short treatment with sleep medication, after consultation with your doctor, if the above tips do not help.

PROVIDE HEALTHYFOOD

Ask your doctor or a dietitian for personal advice to *improve your diet*. The suggestions below will put you on the right path.

- Take your time to enjoy your meals and take them at fixed hours.
- Provide varied and full-fledged nutrition to give your energy level a nice boost.
- Reduce saturated fats, salt and sugar. Thanks to sweetness, your energy level makes a leap forward, but then the bill comes and you go back two steps.

- Avoid products with caffeine. They raise your cortisol level, the stress hormone in your body, which increases your sense of tension.
- Say no to nicotine, stimulant drugs and excessive use of alcohol.
- Avoid ready-made meals.
- Embrace high-fiber foods, vegetables and fruits.
- Drink enough water daily.
- Make sure that eating stays cozy.
- Discover for yourself what your body really needs.
- Do not overdo the adjustments of your diet.
- Eat mindful and be aware of every bite.
- Chew well to improve digestion.

We end with the relationship between stress and certain nutrients.

- Stress steals your B vitamins. Beans, asparagus, peas, mushrooms, brown rice, broccoli, avocados, lentils, eggs, whole grain products, bananas, nuts, seeds and brown rice replenish your stock of B vitamins.
- Because of vitamin C the stress hormone cortisol drops faster in your blood and your immune system is strengthened. Broccoli, peppers, strawberries, watercress, blackberries, tomatoes, citrus fruits and cauliflower are the main suppliers of vitamin C.
- Magnesium has a calming effect on muscles and blood vessels. This substance is found in nuts, especially cashew and almonds, bananas, raisins, avocados, seeds, garlic, seaweed, shellfish, whole grains, quinoa and bitter chocolate.

- Zinc plays an important role in the metabolism and also supports the immune system. Green leafy vegetables, lentils, pumpkin seeds, sesame seeds, almonds, wholegrain cereals and mushrooms are the main providers.
- Omega-3 fats cause an increase of serotonin and give you a more positive state of mind. Eat walnuts, oily fish or flax seeds regularly.

Enjoy your meal!

FOLLOW A BRIAN DIET

Sufficient rest and relaxation, learning to enjoy life, a good night's sleep, healthy food, ... are ideal energy generators to place on your menu.

But if you do not have enough eye for energy wasters, who shamelessly devour your energy, you are talking to a dead phone..

Your brain is the biggest glutton. Your brain accounts for 2% of your body weight, but they do take 20% of your ingested calories. That is why a brain diet - rest assured, you do not have to eat a brain –is indispensable.

If you want to raise your energy level, it is essential to calm your mind and to follow a purification cure.

It is only in the third phase, *the comprehending phase*, that you, with your regained strength, will roll up your sleeves to thoroughly restyle your upper room.

Imagine that your brain has a doorman. Then accept that this doorkeeper has no control over who (= which thought) wants to enter. Do not worry about this! Let it go! You do have authority over who (= what thought) you let in.

At this stage of burnout recovery it is crucial to deny energy wasters access to your life and to offer energy suppliers a VIP card.

There is one person who you should always refuse access. You recognize him directly. He has a T-shirt with the message I MUST. It is anindividual that makes you really tired. Show a bit of understanding for his story, but do not give in and resolutely command him to leave.

We will go deeper into two figures with which your mind often comes into contact:

- incomprehension and expectations of others;
- worrythoughts.

Dealing with incomprehension and expectations of others

Incomprehension usually says nothing about yourself. It is rather a projection of the frustration of someone else.

Where possible, try to promote understanding for your situation. If this turns out not to be achievable, put it in perspective with the thought: "*Everyone has their own limits in terms of empathy!*"

Also, try to turn the lack of empathy in others into an advantage to learn more about yourself. Ask yourself the question "*Do I fully dare to enjoy life while others are at work?*"

If people want to help you with all kinds of well-intentioned invitations, accept that you currently have insufficient petrol in your tank to go into all those invitations. Look at it as an interesting exercise in self-care. Stand up for yourself by, among other things, setting your limits. *No* is even one letter less than *yes*!

Taming your worry head

Why? When? How do I handle this? Your head sometimes looks like a ticket window where screaming teenagers want to get a ticket for the last performance of their idol. Each fan thinks he or she has an acceptable reason to get a ticket. It feels like a torture that you cannot please everyone.

Only 4% of our worry time is about things that affect us. This brings us to the first tip. Arrange all thoughts that bubble in your head according to manageability. Then take the role of doorman again. Only ideas that you have a bit of control over are allowed to enter your brain.

An example to create more clarity! You cannot solve the question "*Why is it raining today?*" This idea is therefore forcefully denied access to your brain. But on the other hand you can handle the question "*How do I ensure that I do not get wet from that rain?*". This thought is allowed free access to your upper room.

Then, in a manner of speaking, it is time to create a sign with '*limited opening hours*' for all those thoughts that you have little or no influence on. During these strictly defined moments - at most half an hour a day - you can convert these thoughts into wishes. The question "*How do I avoid being fired?*" can be changed into the wish "*How do I ensure that I can continue to work in a way that is achievable for me?*"

Outside your opening hours, you kindly point out your thought on the sign with the moments that you are available to them. So your head gets more rest and your energy level is not wasted uselessly.

Time for a second tip! By being focused on quiet and fun activities such as working in the garden, exercising, doing something with a friend, you make your head less accessible to all kinds of questions.

> *"Worrying is fantasizing*
> *in the wrong direction."*
> **- Olaf Hoenson-**

Finally, a selective approach can also help to better control your worry behavior. Limit your thoughts exclusively to the worst case scenario "*What is the worst that could happen?*"

To your own surprise you will perceive that you will often find a solution that is acceptable to you, even for difficult situations like worst case scenarios.

Use this success to suppress the tendency to also examine the other, less severe, scenarios. You have proven to yourself that you will be able to control them if they occur.

Use this strategy to be economical with your thinking energy..

"There are more people who die from worrying than from working,
because there are more people
who are worrying than working."
- based on Robert Frost –

STOP WITH MULTITASKING

We are all over-asked nowadays and try to solve this by tackling several issues at the same time. Even in our free time, it is difficult to escape this. However, research shows that multitaskers are 40% less productive. So immediately *stop multitasking*. It is not profitable because your brain is not equipped for that.

We think we can handle different tasks at the same time, but in reality that is not the case. In reality our brains continuously switch from one activity to another. This requires a lot of brain energy. The result of multitasking is moreover that tasks are often not completed or carelessly finished.

Go for single tasking! Focus on one job and finish it. Do not let yourself be distracted by other issues, such as the phone or your mailbox. If this does happen, learn to become aware of it and congratulate yourself every time you succeed in bringing your attention back to that one task you were working on.

It is more efficient to set priorities and not be distracted by small assignments. In addition, you do well to occasionally free up time to let your thoughts wander and be unreachable. Let your gray mass catch its breath.

Bundling similar assignments is a better alternative if you want to deal with many chores in a short period. This way your focus does not have to change over and over again.

A second option is to call on others. After all, many hands make light work.

LIMIT THE NUMBER OF STIMULI

In our modern society, our brain is stirred up all day by smartphones, e-mails, social media, television, other people's problems, performance pressure, negative thoughts, the busy traffic, ... but above all by being constantly accessible.

Stimuli are sensory impressions that demand your attention. These sensations are part of life, but in our current society they grow even harder than weeds and are equally difficult to exterminate. They cost your body, but especially your upper room, tons of energy.

Because of chronic overstimulation your nervous system gets upset and you become more sensitive to all kinds of impressions. There is over-excitation if more information is received than you are able to process. The result is a long traffic jam in your brain, causing complaints such as concentration problems, mood swings, muscle aches, sleep disturbances, irritation, …

How do you deal with this? The main strategy is to limit stimuli. For example, do not make a call in a room where the radio is on and others have a conversation. Also realize that your body needs time to recover from overstimulation. For example, if you cannot escape a party that feels too busy for you, then allow enough time to relax and recover by staying in a pleasant environment, such as nature.

LIVE A MINDFUL LIFE

Mindfulness is a mindset where you let go of the past and the future. Your mind focuses non-judgmentally on thoughts, feelings and bodily sensations that are exclusively present in the here and now.

Be aware of everything that is happening around you now, but do not delve deeper into it. Do not judge! Observe the surrounding sounds, detect the smells in your vicinity, notice the thoughts that come and go, feel what is happening in your body, … This focus on the present brings deep rest and reduces your tension and stress. If you are tempted to judge, be kind to yourself and do not condemn yourself, but invite yourself to quietly return to the mindfulness mode.

The past and the future are like magnets. They kidnap you from the present. Mindfulness can free you from their grip and bring you back to the here and now.

As you have already experienced several times during your visit to this exhibition, a problem can suddenly cut away the grass under your feet. It seems as if your life and that obstacle coincide. Unconsciously you feel like a photographer who zooms in on that difficulty with his lens, so that the rest of the world apparently disappears.

Mindfulness can help you escape that stranglehold. Use your five senses - *hear, feel, smell, taste and see* - to take in your surroundings and see how the miracle of mindfulness is taking place.

Your life becomes broader. Your camera will zoom out. The problem is not gone and is also not denied, but does shift to the background and is therefore less intense. The stranglehold slaps and you get more space.

> *"Mindfulness is throwing overboard*
> *the past and the future*
> *as feed for the sharks*
> *and throwing the anchor*
> *to pray in the present*
> *without judgment.."*
> **- Don Key -**

Through mindfulness you can distance yourself from problems, automatic reactions, stuck convictions, forced opinions of others, ... You end up in a judgment-free world. This alone is a relief.

Giving conscious judgment-free attention to the here and now is a foundation of mindfulness. Your horse's glasses, your narrowed look full of stereotypical views, will be replaced by a panoramic view that gives you a broad and non-judgmental view of your current existence.

This creates a favorable breeding ground for original insights. Your thinking becomes more creative and you discover other hiking trails for you mind. Your problem solving ability gets a boost and pushes its boundaries.

Mindfulness is a method that you can learn with the intention that it evolves over time into an automatic attitude of life.

TASTE GRATITUDE AND
DISCOVER NOW-HAPPINESS

We interrupt our tour for a sanitary break. I take this opportunity to introduce my d-book, *my gratitude book*, to you. It is a sort of diary in which I write down what I am grateful for in my life. It is not just about moments of happiness. At difficult moments, for example, I can also be grateful for the help I receive or for the interesting life lessons where obstacles make me aware of.

I write briefly, usually at night, for what I have been grateful the past day or I stick a picture in my d-book as a symbol for something that has positively affected me.

Do a little experiment with me! Name five things for what you can be grateful today. Below is my list from yesterday.

- I drank delicious fresh soup.
- I enjoyed an exciting mountain stage during the Tour de France.
- It was a beautiful summer day.
- I have not suffered from physical ailments.
- I have had support from someone when I had a hard time.

You see it: they are not earth-shaking events, but small moments of now-happiness.

Gratitude is a fantastic medicine to combat stress. It has a strong link with mindfulness, because the experience takes place in the present. You can call it now-happiness. This form of prosperity is completely different from goal-happiness, where you first have to achieve something before you can feel good.

With now-happiness you focus on everything that is present in your life and for what you can be grateful. That list is inexhaustible provided that you also mention subjects that seem obvious, such as living in a house, having enough food to live, enjoying nature, drinking water, ...

Self-evidence is often the big bogeyman in our current society. We find so many things normal that we rarely talk about them or are aware of their influence on our sense of happiness. Because of this we do not realize enough what our real wealth is! The more we find everything evident, the smaller becomes the world for which we can be grateful and show admiration.

You also need to take care of everything you already have. What you cherish - certainly do not forget yourself - and treat with respect, increases in value. Wealth has not so much to do with possessions as with appreciating what you have and are grateful for.

In our disposable society we learn that everything is replaceable. Because of this we attach less to things and even persons, which reduces everything in meaning and in value. The pain of the loss decreases, but we do pay a high price: *superficial happiness*.

Now-happiness is always present in the background. It only needs consciousness to establish a connection. A flower, for example, can only give a feeling of happiness if you look at it and give it a moment of awareness. Goal-happiness, on the other hand, has yet to be created. This can cause stress if you doubt the feasibility.

In addition, now-happiness is less intense, but has a longer duration than goal-happiness. It is a feeling of satisfaction, peace with yourself and with the situation in which you find yourself. Now-happinessis inside you as an inexhaustible source. Goal-happiness is more like being flooded by a powerful shower, until the water suddenly runs out.

Gratitude must therefore be practiced consciously, it has to be trained. It is a special way of giving happiness to others, but also to yourself. It works like a boomerang. You pay attention to all the positive things in the present and you are rewarded with a wonderful feeling of happiness. Thanks to gratitude you are no longer dependent on successes and compliments from others for your daily happiness. What a liberation!

By saying thanks for example at the beginning of a meal, by discovering opportunities for appreciation in relationships, ... gratitude becomes the common thread in your life. Thanks to gratitude you also train yourself in viewing the world differently. Your attention focuses more on possibilities than on obstacles.

Also mindfulness can help you with developing gratitude, because this attitude invites you to look at life without judgment. So there is never a feeling of shortage. You are grateful for what is there, even for raindrops!

Some people find it difficult to be grateful. In order to be grateful, you need a positive sense of self-worth. Finding yourself worthwhile is necessary to receive and to be grateful for what is out there, to connect with people, businesses, values, ... If you close yourself to people and things, then there is little to be grateful for.

Make now-happiness the basic foundationfor your life and consider goal-happiness as an extra fountain that you occasionally drink from.

MAINTAIN GOOD SOCIAL CONTACTS

Nice relationships mean enormous support to combat stress and prevent burnout. This includes work relationships such as colleagues, managers, ... and private contacts such as family, family, neighbors, acquaintances, ...

To achieve this, you need to ensure a good balance between work and private life. This will free up enough time to build up and maintain social contacts. For example, systematically doing office work at home is not conducive to the relationship with your partner, children, friends and family.

The sense of belonging gives a good feeling and provides us a more positive self-image. Virtual contacts through social media like Facebook, for example, usually lack the depth we really desire.

If you feel excluded or ignored, it has a profound, negative impact on your well-being. Try to talk about this by indicating how you feel without blaming anyone. Research shows that having a good social network contributes as much to good health as daily physical activity, healthy food, limiting stimulants, etc.

We are happy to help you with some valuable tips to build, maintain and expand a social network.

- Ensure a good balance between work and private life.
- Do not neglect your previous contacts if your circle of acquaintances becomes wider.

- Realize that the development of a social network requires effort and time.
- Dare to show your emotions. It makes you more authentic.
- Show your limits and respect the space of others.
- See to it that your contacts are varied: sometimes listening, offering help, appreciating each other, respecting different points of view, ...

Realize that your partner, family and/or family members, but also your friends, acquaintances and colleagues sometimes feel uncomfortable and powerless in dealing with someone who has a burnout.

Try to clarify what you need, for example a good conversation or just someone to take a walk with.

Do not bypass the hot issues. Bring up where you are not yet ready for, even if the help is well meant, what annoys you, what you are afraid of, what you are angry about, ...

People who want to help somebody with a burnout can use the suggestions below.

- Burnout is a complex issue. Study this subject a bit in order to better understand how far-reaching a burnout can be for someone.
- People with a burn-out can, usually out of powerlessness, react unreasonably or even aggressively. Therefore, do not taketheirreactions personal.

- Find support for yourself and avoid overloading yourself if you are in regular contact with someone who has a burnout.
- Clearly state your own limits with regard to the help you want and can offer to someone with a burnout.

CHOOSE DAILY REGULARITY

What are you doing now with all those energy tips? Make sure that you create regularity and variety in your daily life. On time out of bed, enjoy a quiet breakfast, relax in the shower and occasionally do a light workout, followed by rest. This puts you on the right track to recover from a burnout.

You save energy through a fixed time structure. So you do not have to wonder every day what you will do that day. Create variety: go out with a friend, listen to music, take a short walk, read one chapter from this or another book, visit a museum, explore nature, ...

Provide empty moments in your planning. It is nice to occasionally have time to do something you have not planned. It also gives you a buffer to anticipate on unexpected events in your life.

The guidelines below will provide a daily regularity in your life.

- Do not get up too soon in the morning. Take your time to have breakfast, to take a shower and to get dressed.
- Take a short break after every meal. Your body needs energy for digestion.
- Plan the three meals at fixed times.
- Foresee activities that you like.
- Provide short activities.
- Remember to insert a sport activity every day.
- Always alternate light effort with fun relaxation.
- Provide quiet activities for in the evening.

- Avoid watching TV or working on your computer right before bedtime.
- Go to bed early and stand up without an alarm clock. Only if you have a good night's sleep can you - if you need it - treat yourself to a siesta of 45 minutes in the early afternoon.

BE A GUARD DOG
FOR YOUR ENERGY LEVEL

At the stairs of the next floor we get a drink and we take the time to catch our breath. You receive a notebook from me to write down your daily activities and, with a score of 1 to 5, indicate how high your energy level is when the activity is over.

Following up your activities ensures that you keep an eye on your energy level and adjust where necessary. This should be a way of life to avoid relapse.

We measure the temperature with a thermometer, but how do we determine our energy level? Realize that your energy meter is out of control due to a burnout and no longer works accurately. This needs time to recover.

Because you want to get your life back on track as quickly as possible, there is a big chance of overestimation! After a few weeks of rest you may think that you can go back to work. This is way too early. In the early stages of a burnout your energy tank looks like a box filled with feathers. The box seems full, but when you press on the feathers, you notice that only the bottom is covered.

Take the time you need to fill your energy tank. Only a limited number of people start working after six months. Most people need a year or more to make a new start after a burnout.

COMPREHENCING PHASE

EVALUATE YOUR CURRENT SITUATION

On the second floor we find *the comprehending phase*. The first thing we notice is a large TV screen, on which we immediately recognize the previous floor. This is to point out that the past phase, the charging phase, has not yet been closed. In order to recover from a burnout and to avoid a relapse, it is necessary to keep a close eye on your energy level. This way you can, if necessary, make adjustments in time. Every time we start a new phase, it is important to continue to pay attention to the past periods.

During *the charging phase* you have worked daily to increase your energy level. You now need this fuel to unravel the aspects that play a role in the development, treatment and prevention of burnout.

Your views on how matters relate to each other, for example "*How do I get appreciation from others*" or "*How should I deal with criticism*", have a significant impact on the course of your life and determine whether to develop a burnout.

Stand with a critical eye, without accusing, in front of the mirror. Now examine one by one your predominant beliefs. Discover which ideas, despite good intentions, limit your life.

UNMASK THE MEANING
OF YOUR LIFE

"Why does it get dark? Why do I have to go to bed? Why am I a girl? Why is the grass green? Why whywhy, ...?"

From childhood we ask *'why' questions*. They help us to get a better grip on ourselves, others and the world around us.

"Why do we live?" Is the most popular "why" question that regularly burns on our lips. Behind that question is our need to give meaning to life. The Bushmen speak of two kinds of hunger. The *Little Hunger* listens to the stomach and wants to eat. The *Great Hunger* longs for spirituality.

Life gets meaning when you give meaning to your actions. It is not about what you do, but about why you do something or neglect to do something.

"Man is what he makes of himself
and what he makes of what others think of him.
What you do ultimately shows who you are.
Even if you keep quiet,
your passivity is a form of action.
Your drives give meaning to your actions.
The freedom to create makes you responsible
for your creations, but also for what you do not do."
- based on Jean-Paul Sartre -

Your personality, your identity, is a very dynamic fact. Being is an incessant process of self-realization, in which you determine which needswill receive the most attention. For example, are you someone who focuses primarily on solidarity with others or do you find personal growth more crucial?

"If you lose your identity through your actions,
then you have to stop immediately."
- Stephen King -

You do need a pillar for this enormous building project. Without architect, your life will remain a chaotic construction site.

Parents, teachers, friends, society, your faith, ... are your first support walls. They give you guidance when making decisions. It is your responsibility to gradually take over the task of architect, to draw up and realize an authentic life plan, and where necessary to carry out renovations.

Your life choices are determined by three time questions: "*Who was I? Who am I now? Who can and will I become?*"

Your existence is a balancing act. You sit, as it were, on a seesaw where you can focus on *the 'to-be'-seat* or on *the 'to-become'seat*. In a healthy process of self-realization, '*being*' and '*becoming*' alternate regularly.

When the '*to-be'-chair* is talking:

- then attitudes such as satisfaction and gratitude help you to focus on the positive elements that are there;
- then a mentality of acceptance contributes to letting go of things that you have no control over.

Due to a lack of challenges or due to an excessive urge for certainty, you can stick to the 'to-be'-chair. Then your life seems to stand still. Your existence is burdened with dullness, uselessness, lack of self-confidence, doubts about your own possibilities, denial by pretending to be busy, boredom, indecision, ...

If you have nothing or too little things to do or you do not have enough interests, then you can end up in a bore out. A *bore out* develops in differently than a burnout, but for the rest they both look very similar, because in both cases negative beliefs lead to negative stress.

If, on the other hand, *the 'to-become'-chair* is in charge:

- then attitudes like authenticity, courage and curiosity support you to make new connections;
- then basic attitudes as putting things into perspective, compassion and resilience assist in dealing with disagreements.

If you only aspire *the 'become'-chair*, then you become extinguished, because you do not provide enough time to live in the present. Before you realize it, burnout knocks at your door. Denying, by not opening up, will only aggravate the situation.

The healthy path to self-realization is characterized by a balance between a focus on being and becoming.

DISSOLVE THE ABC-STRESSMODEL

We continue the exhibition and end up in a room that is arranged as a driving school.

Driving school The Full Tank wants to learn people a driving style - lifestyle - while keeping a close eye on their fuel. So they do not end up with an empty tank - a burnout - on the hard shoulder. This is feasible if they are willing to accept certain things in their lives, to change some driving habits and sometimes even to change their route.

We start with the theoretical part of the driving test and show the ABC model of stress and burnout as a reminder.

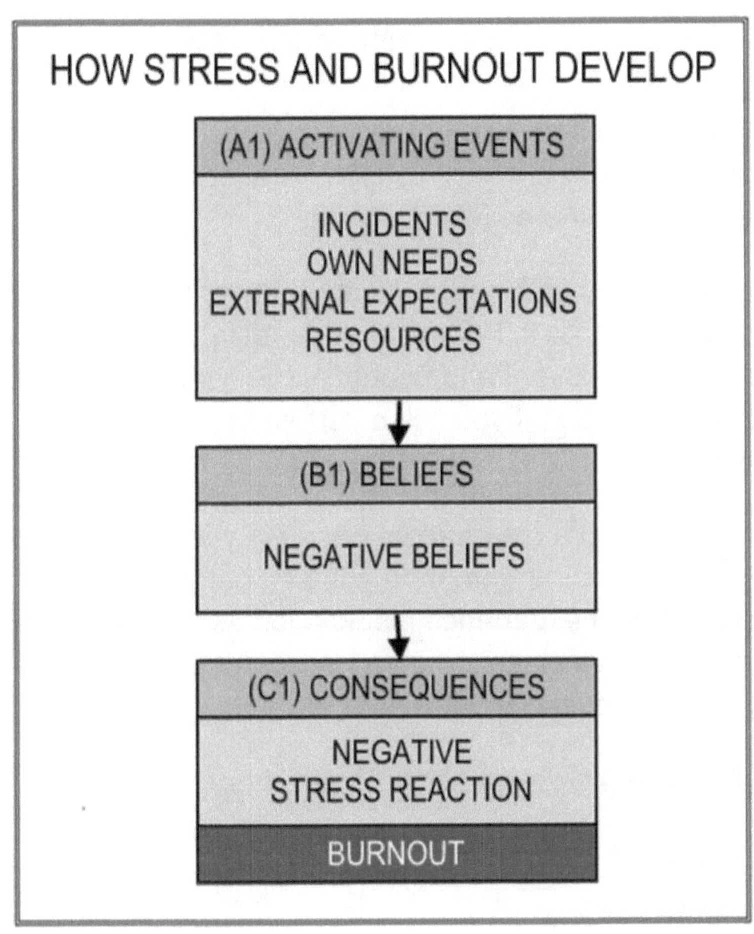

Below we will discuss step by step the various elements that play a role in the development of stress and burnout.

ACTIVATING EVENTS

If you are having a problem or want to realize something, then you usually think in terms of cause and effect. You often forget the first element: the activating event.

An *activating event* is a neutral factor that changes into a cause if you add a belief to it. For example, a resignation is only a neutral activating event and becomes the cause of grief, anger or any other emotion if you link a certain belief to this resignation.

If you do not mind a resignation, because you were already looking out for another job, then you can get the emotion relief as a result. If you experience losing a job as something terrible, because you have plans to buy a house, for example, a feeling of anger may prevail.

We distinguish 4 types of activating events:

- incidents;
- ownneeds;
- external expectations;
- internalandexternal resources.

INCIDENTS

Our lives, both professional and private, are affected daily by all kinds of *incidents* that we have no or little control over. Consider, for example, the resignation of a colleague, a death in the family, rising unemployment, getting a break, the course of your vacation, a rain shower, illnesses, past conflicts at work, initiatives by the government to prevent burnout, ...

It is important to repeat that these incidents have no meaning. They are neutral elements that do not affect your existence. These are factors that, depending on the interpretation you give them, can give rise to a stress response.

People differ from each other in the things they experience and in the belief (s) they link to the incidents in their lives. One person, for example, finds pay reduction worse than the other.

OWN NEEDS

Your *own needs* can, depending on the value you give them, trigger a stress response. For example, if you have an absolute need for security, you will quickly feel negative stress if situations change.

We all have the same six basic needs that we wish to satisfy. These core needs control our existence. We are busy every day, throughout our live and even at night during our dreams, to fill in these basic needs. They are the motives for doing or avoiding something.

People differ from each other in the way they meet their needs and to the extent that they find some needs more important than others. For example, you can relax with alcohol, but also by reading a book. So the need for safety can ensure that you go to the same campsite every year and hope that your spot of last year will still be free or the need for variation challenges you to look for new places.

Tony Robbins distinguishes the following needs:

- the need for *security and comfort*;
- theneed for*variation*;
- the need to *feel special*;
- the need for *love and connectedness*;
- the need for *personal growth*;
- the need to *contribute to a larger whole*.

Everyone has the same needs, but each makes his own choices as to the order of importance of these basic needs and the strategies to be followed to meet those needs.

However, it is not a complete free choice. We are always under the influence of meaningful others such as family, friends, colleagues, society, ... who put forward their values and norms. In addition, our past also has something to say.

After all, there is no fixed relationship between actions and needs. You can take positive and/or negative actions to meet your needs. By buying a house you can constructively build security, but through extreme control of yourself and others you can destructively try to enforce safety.

Now we will go deeper into these various basic needs.

The need for security and comfort

The *need for safety*, predictability and stability ensures that you try to avoid fear and pain and look for factors that can provide you with guidance, such as religion or appointments.

The *need for comfort* such as shelter, sleep, sex, food, ... can give you safety, joy and enjoyment.

Although it is dangerous to make a statement about what is the most important need, I would like to point out that a considerable dose of stability and predictability is needed to meet the other needs. For example, without basic safety it is impossible to develop healthy relationships.

Beware! Avoid a blind desire for a world with much comfort, complete security and complete manageability, because then feelings like fearfor losing safety and boredom, because there are no challenges, will beon your daily menu.

The need for variation

As soon as a foundation of certainty is present, the need for *variation* and challenges arises. Just think of the exploration drive among young children.

By shifting your physical, emotional and psychic boundaries, you enrich your life. How we fill in our need for variation differs from person to person. One, for example, is looking for different hobbies and the other needs an extensive circle of acquaintances.

Just as with certainty, dosage is also important here. Too much variation and uncertainty about comfort can make you anxious and can be paralyzing. You need a certain degree of safety to enjoy variety.

The need for safety and the need for variation have a kind of yin-yang relationship. The more security and comfort you experience, the greater the urge becomes for more variety and sobriety in your life and vice versa.

The need to feel special

We all feel the need to develop our individuality. We have an innate desire for self-realization. This does not always happen without a struggle. Just think of the endless discussions between young people and their parents about choice of clothing, the cleanliness of their room, the friends they hang out with, ...

Our need for love and connectedness - see the following basic need - can be so persistent that we put too much of our individuality aside to meet the expectations of others. Then the most disturbing conviction of all is created. We think *"I'm not good enough!"* This false belief - which we all more or less suffer of - plays a major role in almost all physical, psychological and emotional problems.

However, if you focus too much on your talents, then there is the danger that you will start to feel better than others. You will then be isolated. This is an obstacle to the following basic need: *the urge for love and solidarity.*

The need for love and connectedness

Everyone is lifelong in *search for love* and feels *the need to be connected* with himself and others.

In your belief system, mistakes can misguide you about your need to give or receive love. So for example you can mistakenly think that you are not good enough to receive love and that you therefore have to do everything perfectly.

The need for love and connection can be so great and seem so unrealizable that there is a danger that you will reach out for unhealthy stimulants such as stealing, drugs, vandalism, alcohol, ... to feel connected to a certain group.

Connection is not limited to persons. You can also feel connected to art, animals, nature or a certain doctrine such as Buddhism, liberalism, ...

The need for personal growth

Everything that lives is characterized by growth. If we do not continue to evolve mentally, emotionally or spiritually, we may feel that we no longer exist. Then it feels as if our life is locked. Standing still can feel like going backwards!

> *"It requires courage to grow and*
> *to become the person you are deep inside."*
> **- E. E. Cummings -**

Our lives require regular maintenance, just like a garden, to continue to grow. You should constantly develop values such as authenticity, gratitude, tolerance, honesty, helpfulness, ... to avoid being overrun by misleading concepts such as power, property, status, ...

Personal growth never retires. If you want to keep your relationships, your body, your finances, your work, ... in good condition, you have to take care of it every day.

The need to contribute to a larger whole

Participating in society, for example by being active in politics, in cultural associations, or by volunteering, gives you a sense of happiness that is of a different quality than the focus on your own life.

Reducing this need has a positive influence on all your other needs. Being able to give gives you certainty. You can give everything: material things, money, attention, love, friendship, forgiveness, ... Variation in abundance! It gives you a feeling of being special and by helping you make a connection with others.

Making a *contribution to a larger whole* gives you a sense of immortality. You grow further in the other and in society by giving something of yourself. This is not limited to material matters. For example, you can be immortalized by writing a book.

"Life is a gift.
It offers you the privilege, the opportunity
and the responsibility

EXTERNAL EXPECTATIONS

Your life revolves around fulfilling your basic needs. To meet these needs as good as possible, it is necessary to find a balance between your desires and *the expectations of others*.

With others we mean people like family, friends, colleagues, neighbors, strangers, ... but also structures like the company where you work, the school of your children, associations of which you are a member, the various authorities, the legislation, religious guidelines, ...

Our environment is changing rapidly and more and more people are struggling to find a place in today's society. It looks like it has been poisoned. If we take a close look at the rising numbers of unemployment, illness, burnout, aging, poverty, ... we get the impression that our modern COBRA-society spits out more and more people with the grounds: *not good enough*.

A COBRA society expects us to be able to deal with Complexity, Overruling personality, Banishing stability, Risk taking and Ambiguity.

We are going to have a close look at these five characteristics and their influence on our well-being.

Dealing with Complexity

The combination of family life and work creates a complex situation. It requires a lot of planning and adjustments to ensure that everything runs smoothly. More and more people become overloaded by deadlines, responsibilities on which they are insufficiently prepared, limited financial resources, little support from third parties and expectations such as almost permanent accessibility and knowledge of new technologies such as the Internet.

Especially the emotional and mental strain increases, because people cannot or do not want to free up enough time to get rid of tension by, for example, exercising or meditating, or just saying no if they are too busy. This often leads to unworkable situations.

Dealing with Overruling personality

Companies find it difficult to approach their staff in a sufficiently personal way by giving them more autonomy and offering adapted work. Employees feel that they are not sufficiently addressed in their unique talents and experience too little recognition and appreciation from their supervisors.

Reorganizations within companies often cause staff turnover which makes it difficult to build social contacts with colleagues.

The rise of e-mail traffic also creates more distance between employees. There is less and less time for a chat at the coffee machine!

Due to busy schedules we run from one appointment to
another. For example, there is no time to catch up after the
yoga class, because you have to pick up the children from the
music class. This makes it difficult to build a supporting social
network.

Dealing with Banishing stability

Mobility is about the speed of changes in our lives. A generation
ago, for example, teaching a profession still provided sufficient
job stability. Our COBRA-society, however, requires lifelong
learning and continuous ability to take on other functions and
responsibilities.

Employees are required to be flexible, also in terms of working
hours, and to adequately anticipate and respond to rapidly
changing situations.

The technology train with smartphones, tablets, e-mails, social
media, scanning devices, ordering online ... demands a high
mobility of its passengers.

Dealing with Risk taking

Due to competitive pressure companies are taking higher risks
with uncertainty as a result. Just think of the stock market crash
and the banking crisis.

Increasing terrorism also causes growing doubt and
unpredictability in our society.

Rising uncertainties with questions like: *"Will there still be a sufficient pension?,What about the stock of fossil fuels?"*, ... make decisions like "*How long will I continue to work?, Which car will I buy?, ... "*increasingly risky.

Dealing withAmbiguity

Our contemporary reality is also characterized by increasing ambiguity. Just look at our legislation and the morality of our society. They are full of ambiguities and contradictions.

Because of the large mobility and complexity of society, companies are increasingly failing. They do not succeed enough to come out with a clear mission and vision.

INTERNAL AND/OR EXTERNAL RESOURCES

To cope with incidents, to meet your own needs and external expectations, you can call in the help of internal and/or external resources.

Examples ofinternal resources

- Your personal skills as acceptance, empathy, daring to show vulnerability, forgiveness, cherishing hope, being patient, showing discipline, showing gratitude, seeing problems as challenges, being able to specify limits,

dealing with criticism, asking for help, taking distance, indicate how you feel and how you think, ...
- Your life and work experiences. This concerns both the positive and negative issues that you have experienced.
- The absence of serious difficulties such as alcoholism, sleep problems, serious illnesses, loneliness, ...
- Your self-image, the image you have of others and of society.
- Your work and/or life experience.
- ...

Examples ofexternal resources

It concerns resources in the private as well as in the work situation.

- Clarity of jobdescription.
- Amount of duties and workload.
- Freedomto act.
- Opportunities for personal development.
- The extent to which you receive appreciation and remuneration.
- Job security and/or life stability.
- Work and/or living environment.
- The attention you get for your well-being.
- Communication structures.
- Relationships withothers.
- ...

Internal and external resources only support you if you actually see them as help. For example, a colleague becomes a

resource only if you give him or her that label and allow his or
her support.

NEGATIVE BELIEFS

As you already know, activating events are neutral elements.
They have no meaning and therefore no direct impact on your
life. Only when give them a specific label they will influence your
existence. Then you can get beliefs like "*My boss checks me
because he does not trust me enough.*" or "*The extra work is
too stressful and does not give me satisfaction, because I have
to justify every decision.*"

These beliefs govern your life and have important
consequences. They are responsible for the type of stress you
experience, your emotional life, your physical sensations such
as upset stomach and the actions you take or avoid.

> *"There is no good or bad,*
> *but thinking creates it!"*
> **- William Shakespeare -**

Fortunately, not every belief gets a negative label. We will
briefly discuss the different types of beliefs that you can create.

<u>Types of beliefs</u>

We distinguish four possible beliefs in response to an activating event. For example, how can we respond to the activating event '*extra work*'?

- *Positive*: you like the extra work. It finally gives you the chance to show your talents.
- *Negative*: you find it disturbing that there is more work. You're already so busy.
- *Irrelevant:* you do not mind that the work increases. You will, in one way or another, ensure that your workload will not be increased as a result.
- *Ambiguous:* the extra work has both advantages and disadvantages for you.

You notice once again that judging is a very subjective issue. There are no absolute facts, but only the attribution of personal truth labels.

> *"Truth is the name we give*
> *to changing mistakes."*
> **- Rabindranath Tagore -**

We deliberately used the same factor - extra work - as an example. This is to show that your belief and not the activating events determine how you experience something.

NEGATIVE CONSEQUENCES

If you connect activating events, such as getting an assignment, with false beliefs, such as "*I may not fail if my boss comes up with a new assignment*", then you end up in a state of negative stress. Then your false beliefsare the real cause of your negative stress.

Because of negative stress self-realization, your overarching goal of life is jeopardized. It is a fact that due to the strong unpleasant emotions and the inefficient actions that you undertake as a result of the stress, you are unable to neutralize the negative stress and avoid burnout.

How is this process now in detail?

NEGATIVE STRESS

Stress puts you in a higher state of readiness. It gives you the strength and the alertness you need to react appropriately in (life) threatening situations. This safety mechanism is automatically triggered as a result of circumstances that your body considers to be highly deviant. Stress in itself is not negative or positive.

We use the term negative or positive stress when we want to draw attention to the possible consequences. If the physical sensations and the emotions as a result of stress, allow you to take effective actions, which takes you a step further on your path to self-realization, then there is positive stress. In the other case, we experience negative stress and can eventually end up in a burnout.

NEGATIVE ACTIONS

You may think, feel and plan as much as you like, but only actions can lead to a real change.

"Happiness comes from your own actions."
- Dalai Lama XIV -

You can approach an obstacle in different ways. For example, you can take a walk when you are angry, you may postpone a difficult task until tomorrow, you can ask others for help, ... Everyone learns methods during their life to deal with obstacles and reduce stress. These methods are called *coping styles*.

Coping includes our intellectual and/or behavioral efforts to tackle, mitigate and/or (partially) accept stress. Usually your approach consists of various coping tactics. The choice for one or more strategies to deal with a particular stress factor is related to previous experiences and your courage to tolerate unpleasant physical sensations and emotions.

If you are in a state of negative stress, your room for maneuver will be limited to four coping methods.

We distinguish: *avoiding obstacle*, *minimizing difficulty*, *overcompensating malfunctions* and *looking at the situation passively*.

These tactics bring relief in the short term, but cannot solve the situation for the future and sometimes even aggravate it.

- ***Avoiding obstacle***
  - *Distraction*: you seek distraction by, for example, walking instead of arranging your administration.
  - *Denial*: you do not take any action, for there is nothing to worry about according to you.
  - *Postponing*: you think of reasons such as "*It heals automatically*", in order not to go to the doctor.
  - *Withdrawing*: for example, you watch excessive TV with the excuse that you like to be alone or you take psychological distance by living in a dream world.
  - *Looking for tension*: you compensate for your difficult situation by, for example, practicing extreme sports like bungee jumping.
  - *Numb*: for example, you relax yourself through alcohol, drugs, excessive food, ...

- ***Minimizing difficulty***
  By minimizing and explaining away you fool yourself that the incident is not so bad: "*It will be okay, others have also experienced this*", ... You are creating reassuring thoughts.

- ***Overcompensating malfunctions***
  - *Hostility*: you counterattack by for example accusing your boss of unreasonableness. This can also happen (passively) by sabotaging the situation sneakily. For example, you accidentally arrive late again.

- o *Search for self-confirmation*: for example, you set the bar extremely high for yourself to impress others.
  - o *Manipulate*: for example, you try to control the situation through deception.
  - o *Exaggerated actions*: you attempt, for example by obsessively following the rules, to show that you are not the cause.

- **Looking at the situation passively**
  - o *Compliance*: you avoid conflicts and behave submissively.
  - o *Depressive reactions*: you blame yourself, you worry a lot, you doubt your possibilities, ...

If you are aware of the coping strategies that you apply, you are well on the right track. Breaking patterns is often very difficult and takes a lot of time. We will come back to this later.

BURNOUT

If your actions do not lead to a desirable result, the negative stress will continue to increase. When it reaches a too high level, is constantly present in your life and is not properly addressed by you, your body remains in imbalance for too long and a dangerous condition of chronic negative stress arises.

This situation, which can lead to a burnout, can be recognized by increasing physical, psychological, emotional and behavioral complaints.

<u>**Recognizable physical complaints**</u>

- Persistent fatigue.
- Insomnia.
- Muscle pain, headache, neck pain, back pain, ...
- Stomach pain, intestinal disorders, poor appetite, ...
- Reducedresistancetoinfections.
- Palpitations and / or tension on the chest.
- Difficultbreathing.
- The feeling of fainting.
- Sweatingandclammy hands.
- Changingappetiteandweight.
- Raisedbloodpressure.
- Increased cholesterol levels.
- ...

<u>**Typical psychological and emotional symptoms**</u>

- No more peace of mind, agitation, ...
- Irritable or irritated.
- Gloomy showers, crying, worrying, fear, ...
- No more enjoyment, being lethargic and lifeless.
- Indecision, loss of concentration, forgetfulness, ...
- Feeling of meaninglessness of life.
- Negativism, cynicism, being more critical, ...
- Uncertainty, lessself-confidence, ...
- Quicklydistractedandscattered.
- Reducedability torelativize.
- ...

Representativebe havioral characteristics

- Perform less (fast) and make more mistakes.
- Use more smoking, alcohol or drugs.
- Taking refuge in sleeping and tranquilizers.
- Increasedunhealthydietaryhabits.
- Lesscreativityandperseverance.
- Being inclined to flee work and/or relationships.
- Automatic actions become more difficult.
- …

Too often people underestimate stress phenomena and think that the storm will also blow over. The reverse is usually true. It often evolves from bad to worse.

Due to a long overdose of stress, people become overwrought and physically, psychologically and emotionally exhausted.

Ordinary everyday tasks gradually become inadmissible obstacles. Even rest and relaxation prove to be insufficient to turn the tide. Due to the accumulation of all kinds of problems you can get a burnout. Your effective actions then take off and due to self-protection you distance yourself psychologically and emotionally frompeople, your tasks, your living situation and your environment. You also doubt your own coping skills.

In a situation of excessive stress and overload, there is still a commitment to achieve objectives. The inability in you to reverse the situation in a positive direction is growing and leaves deep psychological and emotional traces. You have some hope, but you live on adrenaline. You tell yourself that you have everything under control and you try to solve the problem by boosting your efforts. Without drastic changes, overload will end in a burnout.

When you have a burnout, you still want to achieve things, but you do not succeed anymore. Your tank is completely empty. Your feelings become flattened. You also psychically distance yourself from your responsibilities. You feel helpless and left to your fate. Life escapes you. You undergo your situation and no longer take any initiatives. The quality of your work, both private and professional, becomes insufficient. You end up in a negative spiral that further intensifies the negative stress resulting in a burnout.

It is time to address this negative stress!

ATTACK NEGATIVE STRESS
AND BURNOUT

We have arrived at the most important part of the exhibition: *tackling and avoiding negative stress, in order to neutralize burnout and pave the way to self-realization.*

If you are exposed to unhealthy stress for a long period, you will not succeed sufficiently in fulfilling your basic needs in dialogue with your environment. From your basic needs an underground resistance grows, a protest voice that says: "*I do not want to live like that anymore!*" Burnoutforces you to listen to your inner voice.

Burnout puts your life on a chain with a special lock. Desperately, you try to free yourself with your familiar old keys, such as taking a break, doing your best, even harder ... but in vain. Only when you realize that you need new keys, then you really understand what burnout wants to tell you.

Incidents, for example a disease, limited resources, for example an unclear organization, or external expectations, for example a high workload, can cause a growing overload. However, the negative beliefs, convictions that you ironically created yourself, are the culprits making it difficult to get you out of this impasse.

As a coach of your own life you carry the primary responsibility to change strategy in time. It is your job to ensure that you do not lose your life match. You can achieve this by removing negative beliefs from the field and by giving confidence to disowned and hidden beliefs that are positive and have been waiting impatiently for a chance to show their talents.

"*I am good enough*" is the positive belief with the highest scoring power. This belief should become the mantra of your team. Also, ideas like "*I can make a mistake*" and "*Setbacks are part of life*" deserve a basic place in your life team.

Below you will find the ABC-scheme with steps of treatment and prevention in case of negative stress and burnout.

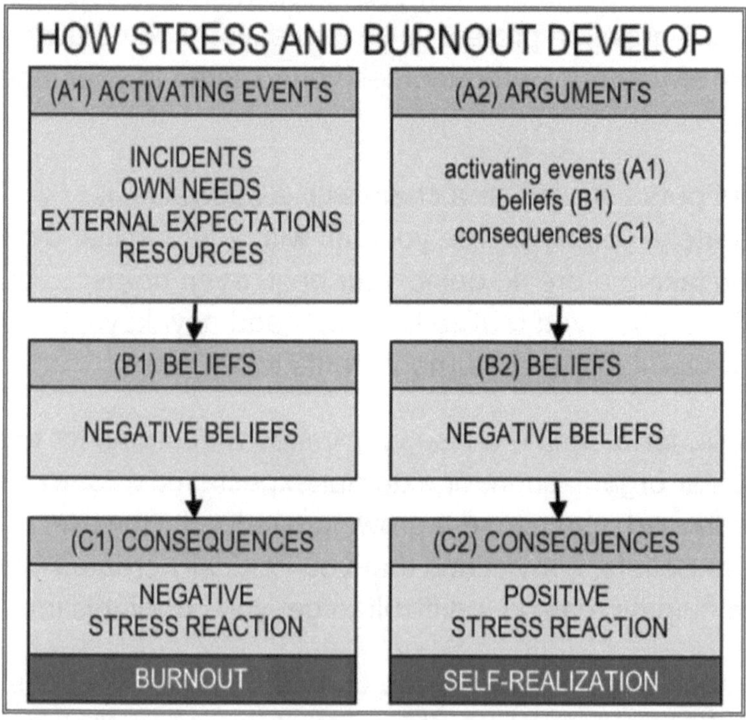

How do you deal with negative stress? We opt for a tactic with three pillars:

- dismantle the ABC-stress factors (= activating events, beliefs and consequences) with arguments;
- learn more about negative beliefs;
- develop positive actions.

To dismantle the ABC-stressfactors you can fall back on:

- experience questions;
- logicalquestions;
- practical questions.

More about this later!

DISMANTLE THE ABC-STRESSFACTORS

For our approach and prevention of stress and burnout, we got the inspiration from the RET therapy of Albert Ellis (1913-2007).

According to this method, stress and burn-out result from incorrect observations of activating events and wrong interpretations (= negative beliefs) of the situation in which you find yourself. As a result, you are a crucial factor in the emergence of negative stress and burn-out. On the other hand this has the plus point that you are in control to bend the situation to your advantage.

*"The biggest part of what we call personality
is determined by how we have chosen
to defend ourselves against problems."*
- by Alain de Botton-

Our approach and prevention of stress and burnout include:

- contradict activating events with arguments;
- contradict beliefs with arguments;
- contradict consequences with arguments.

You will investigate whether the arguments you have used to treat activating events, beliefs and consequences as causal elements of your stress and burnout are correct and complete.

CONTRADICT ACTIVATING EVENTS

How objective is your image of the reality in which you live? To observe *activating events* (A) without prejudices, you need to look at incidents, own needs, external expectations and resources as if you were the lens of a camera.

A camera does not record emotions, but only faithfully observes reality. How quickly do we say, for example, "*I saw him staring at me suspiciously.*" Then realize that only the word 'looking' is objective. The addition 'suspiciously' is a subjective interpretation. 'Staring' is also subjective, because it refers to a certain way of perception. Even 'to me' is not objective. Maybe he was looking at someone behind me that I was not aware of.

Realize that complete objectivity is not feasible. Too many things happen in your environment and your senses also have their limitations in perceiving.

Try to search for more objectivity through the questions below.

- Wat zie ik werkelijk en wat is een interpretatie? Zie ik bijvoorbeeld mijn collega een hand geven aan de baas of zie ik hem/haar slijmen met de baas?
- What do I really see and what is an interpretation? Do I see my colleague shaking hands with the boss or do I see him / her slimming with the boss?
- What do I want to achieve? Do I want to increase my talents, for example, or do I want to impress others?

CONTRADICT BELIEFS WITH ARGUMENTS

As you know by now, finding arguments to neutralize negative beliefs is your main weapon to reduce stress and avoid burnout.

*"Our greatest weapon against stress isour ability
to choose one thought over another."*
- William James -

For the sake of clarity we repeat that we can divide beliefs into two groups..

- *Negative beliefs*: these are views, such as "*I am not allowed to fail*", which paralyze you and prevent you from living a happy life.

- *Positive beliefs*: these are ideas, such as "*I love myself*", that make you more resilient, so that you can deal better with setbacks and show you the way to a fuller existence.

It often happens that positive beliefs, through the power of negative opinions, fade into the background or never see the light of day. So the statement "*A good collegial atmosphere is important*" must then put the thumbs for the idea "*Atmosphere is subordinate to results*".

Your treasure chest with *disowned and hidden beliefs* possesses the power to push the *ruling, negative beliefs* of their throne and thus turn your life in a more positive direction.

"The key to insight
lives in each of us."
- Tao Meng-

In the *commitment phase*, during the workshop *'Convince yourself of new beliefs'*, we search for the key, the key to open this treasure chest. Then you will find a beautiful pearl necklace with sparkling, disowned and hidden beliefs to address your stress.

How did negative beliefsbecome successful in attracting power?

Negative beliefs have carried out a ruthless advertising campaign and have succeeded in being purchased by you. They have touted themselves with sales arguments such as "*I am the only right one, it is right, this gives absolute safety, that's how you get appreciation, now you're fully involved, ...*"

These obstructing beliefs are cunning guys who have managed to convince you of their qualities. They have settled in your headquarters and have been crowned as the management committee of your personality. These crafty rascals have managed to force a high credit rating and mask their dark sides.

Because you believe them, they become your truth. Now the are in charge and do not tolerate participation. They determine who you are, what you think, feel and do.

But, what is even important: they also decide '*who you are not allowed to be, what you should not think, feel and do*'! That way they shape your identity. Fear is their strongest weapon to restrain you.

> *"Overcoming fear is breaking the shell*
> *that opens up the insight of your inner wisdom."*
> **- based on Kahlil Gibran -**

In order to avoid a burnout, to recover from it or to prevent relapse, it is confrontational, but necessary, to get to know your predominantbeliefs. Restrictive ideas have the following recognizable characteristics.

Negative beliefs are often:

- *demanding*: you have to do this, it is not allowed to do that ... Think for example of the thought "*I want people to like me and that's why they should like me*";
- *extreme*: it is terrible that, it is disastrous that, it is unacceptable that, ... For example, you have the way of thinking "*It is absolutely terrible when people come late*";

- *intolerant*: it bothers me, it is annoying that, ... For example, you hear the statement: "*I can not stand it when people quarrel*";
- *(self)judgmental*: if you fail, you are weak; if you rest, then you are lazy; ... Perhaps you sometimes use the conviction "*If people find me unkind, then I'm not good enough*";
- *comparative*: the others will think that, ... Some people, for example, use the idea "*If I make a mistake, they will find me stupid*";
- *Anxiety-inducing*: if you do not do this, then ... You may be bothered by the statement "*If I do not check everything carefully, then it's my fault if something goes wrong.*"

Finally, we often mistakenly think that our beliefs are effective if they contain a positive message and vice versa, but that factor is not decisive. The idea "*I always have to be ready for everyone*" is positive, for example, but ineffective because of the extreme character (always /everybody).

CONTRADICTING CONSEQUENCES

Finally, you will tackle the consequences. You reflect on the sensations, feelings and behaviors that you actually desire.

"Happy people plan actions."
- Denis Waitley -

Through a step-by-step plan you can find out which positive, hidden or disowned beliefs you need to get from under the dust.

In the example below, you try to come up with the positive beliefs that are needed to create the emotions you want to feel more often, for example *'pride'*.

- For example, make contact with the emotion '*being proud of yourself*'.
- Look for a belief that helps to cause this feeling. Consider, for example, the statement "*I am a go-getter.*"
- Think of additional beliefs that you can use to reinforce this feeling. For example, what do you think of the thought "*If I compare with the past, I can now sing, dance better*"?
- Breathe quietly and deeply, let the positive beliefs do their work and smile at yourself.
- Feel how everything slowly becomes calmer.
- Keep up with this technique.

COME UP WITH QUESTIONS
TO FIND ARGUMENTS

You can come up with various questions to find arguments with which you can neutralize activating events (A), negative beliefs (B) and disruptive consequences (C).

For this you can use experience questions, logical questions and practical questions.

<u>**Experience questions**</u>

In case of experience questions you will, just like a public prosecutor, look for evidence. Which arguments can I find pro and contra?

You can use the following questions for this.

- Is it true that...? Is it right, for example, that I am always bullied by everyone?
- Where is the evidence that ...? Where, for example, is proof that my boss never gives me a compliment?
- Can I demonstrate that these activating events are correct? Can I prove, for example, that I never have time to take a short break?

<u>**Logical questions**</u>

If you are dealing with if-then arguments, it is advisable to check whether one thought logically follows the other.

Here you will find the following types of questions.

- Is it true that if ... then ... must? Is it correct, for example, that I always get the biggest assignment if there is extra work?
- Does one result in the other? For example, is my fatigue due solely to the amount of work?
- Do I always have the experience that if ... then ... must? Do I find, for example, that I always have to say 'yes' when a colleague asks me for help?

<u>**Practical questions**</u>

For practical questions you study the effect on your life. What does this mean for my feelings, thoughts and behaviors?

You can use the questions below.

- Do I wish ...? Do I find it important, for example, to get challenging assignments?
- Does this idea help me to feel ...? Will I feel proud if, for example, I think I can organize well?

DISCOVER THE MAIN NEGATIVE BELIEFS

Your *beliefs* (B) are your most formidable opponents. Try to undermine the validity of your prevailing opinions with arguments. If you can floor them, you have a great chance to prevent or reduce negative stress and burnout. For example, you can minimize the belief "*Everything has to go perfectly*" with the argument "*If I do not mind making mistakes, I will have less stress.*"

We will run through the main obstructing beliefs that hinder people in their path to self-realization.

<u>**Everyone should like and respect me**</u>

This is an illogical idea, because it means that everyone would think the same way. It is more rational to accept that there will always be people who do not like you because they have a different opinion about what is more or less important or what is acceptable and what is not.

You realize this by interpreting the reactions of others in the following way: "*What people think about me only says something about what they find important, but says nothing about me as a person. Afterall, we are all a mirror for each other!* "

Imagine it is achievable and everyone loves you. This may seem like heaven on earth, but actually you are now in the trap. In order to maintain this situation, you may not commit any missteps. You should always be reasonably, socially and positively oriented. What a stifling corset! A real hell, if you ask me.

It is advisable to investigate whether there might be a misunderstanding that makes people find you unkind. You can simply check this by asking yourself: "*Do I understand you correctly that you think that ...?*"

Pleasers often suffer from this belief. They hope to be liked by others because of their helpfulness. Out of fear of rejection, they quickly seek a compromise in case of problems, because they want to avoid the difficult emotions of a conflict. Usually pleasers give too much ground. Of course you do not have to provoke conflicts unnecessarily, but a collision sometimes creates more clarity and sometimes opens up new solution paths.

Moreover, pleasers recognize their own pains, disappointments, frustrations and fears in other persons. By pleasing others, they try to alleviate their own suffering and grief.

If I make a mistake, then I am worthless

This belief leads to perfectionism and fear of failure. Especially linking performance to self-worth ensures that you put yourself under enormous pressure. In extreme cases, situations such as misunderstandings, setbacks, distractions are also considered as personal failures.

Accept that you, just like everyone else, have limits. Tune your goals to your own capabilities.

"In life you do what you can,
but what you want is not always feasible."
- motto of my 80-year-old mother -

On the other hand if something does not go as planned, then it makes sense to find out whether it is possible to avoid this in the future.

By constantly pushing your boundaries, stress increases and your fear of failure is fed. Moreover, there is a real chance that you also want others to be perfect, so as a result you will be regularly confronted with disappointments and frustrations.

The following statements, to a greater or lesser extent, apply to perfectionists.

- They need others to confirm that they are valuable.
- They set the performance bar high for themselves and for others.
- They are dissatisfied with their actions and assume that they do not meet the expectations of others.
- They need the feeling of control and hope to find peace in this way.
- They are often on the lookout to keep an eye on everything. The focus is on what can fail and not on what is okay and has a chance of success.
- They have problems with making decisions, because they may make the wrong choices.
- They feel guilty quickly, because everything that goes wrong, they judge as a personal failure.
- They go beyond their own limits and also put pressure on other people to do the same.

Perfectionists are workaholics with a crowded agenda and their day is often too short. They are restless, tense, impatient and very task-oriented. Because of that tension, they regularly show strong emotional reactions, even on small, innocent stimuli.

Bad people must be punished

You know them, 'colleagues who only do the much-needed and do not receive any comments about their minimalist attitude'. And if in addition you are not appreciated for your extra efforts, then you are completely disappointed. You find it inadmissible that people who neglect their duties are not tapped on their fingers.

The fallacy often committed here is condemning people as a person on the basis of their

It is more correct to accept that people have built up their own hierarchy of values and norms through their culture, upbringing and experiences. Who are we to set our standards above those of others?

If we show sufficient tolerance, we can deal more easily with people who have different policies.

I can not stand it if things do not go as I want

This is about acceptance. If we get annoyed quickly if people do not respond as we like or if things do not go as planned, we have a low frustration tolerance threshold. We do not need much to end up in a bad mood.

Setbacks and oppositions are inevitable ingredients of everyone's existence. Make sure your reaction does not aggravate the situation. For example, people who are stuck in a traffic jam do not move faster by getting angry.

It is more sensible to check how setbacks have arisen. This will allow you to avoid problems in the future. But you also have to accept that bad luck can never be completely eliminated from your life and that there will always be uncertainties that you can only accept.

It is never up to me if things go wrong

Some people find that the cause of problems always lies with someone else or in external circumstances that they have no control over. Such persons crawl into a victim role. They take insufficient action to tackle the situation and avoid their own responsibility.

This is too extreme attitude. You do have a certain degree of influence on the direction of your life river, but sometimes you have to swim against the current. It does require a realistic assessment of your possibilities and limitations. For such people it remains a challenge to find their way in such situations.

I must always be prepared for misery

People with this belief are living in fear all the time. The danger lurks, according to them, around every corner. They also think that everyone wants to disadvantage them.

Pessimists repeatedly display ineffective behavior, which regularly causes what they are afraid of. This way they are confirmed in their premonitions. This common mechanism is known under the name *self-fulfilling prophecy*.

One approach that can help is the *worst case scenario strategy*. You then hypothetically dwell on the worst that can happen to you and then imagine the best approach for this. You will notice that even for the worst things, of which you are not sure that they will happen, you can often think of an acceptable tactic.

Try to draw enough confidence from this, so that it is unnecessary to spend time analyzing other things that might go wrong.

Encourage yourself with the thought "I have found an acceptable solution for the worst case scenario, so I will know how to handle things that I have not prepared for."

I am completely dependent on others

By asking others for advice on each assignment or decision, you make it impossible to build your self-esteem and to be valued and respected by others.

As social beings, it is normal and appropriate that we ask each other for support and help, but nobody benefits from complete dependence.

Look at your relationships with others on a regular basis and ask yourself what more independence would mean for your self-confidence and for your self-respect. A cake with, for example, a strange shape can give you a good feeling if you do not focus on the view, but on the fact that you have baked it yourself and that it tastes good.

My life is mainly determined by my past

This is a very negative thought. You've certainly already heard the verdict "*I am who i am based on everything I've experienced. There is nothing more to change.*"

Because of this idea people no longer believe in opportunities for change in themselves and others. They settle for fate, but do not realize that they themselves create this fate through their opinions.

Of course we are influenced by the past, and drastic events can still have a strong impact on the present, but thanks to time, acceptance and, above all, making new choices, old wounds can soften and fixed patterns can be broken.

I have to help people who are in need

This claim is mainly about the motive used for helpfulness. Many people are concerned about others and try to conceal in such a way that they are unable to master their own difficulties or they exhibit this behavior because they do not find themselves good enough.

The great danger with this impeding conviction is that you take over the responsibility of the other person. This is disastrous for the self-confidence of that other person. Dosage is also indicated here.

I have to find the best solution for each problem

It is the reality that for many problems there is only a limited solution or sometimes even no suitable outcome can be imagined.

This disturbing beliefs ensures that people remain stuck in a decision process for too long, resulting in procrastination. They tend to postpone tackling a problem for themselves. They feed on the thought "*If I do nothing, I will not do anything wrong.*"

Procrastination often causes difficulties to get worse and you will no longer see the trees through the forest. Extra work is created through memories or forgotten and delayed assignments. A useful tip: start every day with something you do not like. Willpower is a muscle that gets stronger through daily training.

Avoiding responsibilities is a risky choice. In time, your self-image will become increasingly negative and your self-confidence will drop below freezing. You will hate yourself because you start to believe less in your own competences.

The resilience that you need to tackle problems also drops to an all-time low. Moreover, such an attitude is not welcomed by applause by your environment, so isolation becomes a real danger.

Consider obstacles as a challenge to show yourself and others what you are capable of. Focus,if you judge yourself, especially on the way you approached and addressed the situation. Less attention to the result, because you never 100% in the hand.

First determine for yourself what an acceptable outcome is,
even if it is not ideal. Then look for the best solution and apply it.

You can try other things afterwards, but it is important that you
also limit this, at a certain moment you must be satisfied with
what you have achieved and accept what has not been
successful.

"You're only human after all."
- based on Daft Punk -

DEVELOP POSITIVE ACTIONS

By neutralizing negative beliefs and creating positive beliefs,
you are now in a state of positive stress.

The tension that you feel is stimulating. You are challenged to
tackle the problem and you have sufficient confidence in your
chances of success.

The physical sensations and the feelings are not always
pleasant, but they are never so obstructive that they have a
paralyzing effect and prevent you from creating and setting up
positive actions.

If you have a hard time, look for additional positive statements
to stimulate yourself and investigate if there are no negative
beliefs that are foolishly misleading your brain.

It is difficult to clearly determine the best approach to combat stress. We can however indicate which factors play a significant role in this decision-making process.

The following questions will help you on your way.

- *Do I have control over the situation?*In every stressful context, the choice of your actions depends on the degree to which you feel you have control or not. Do you think, for example, that people will follow your advice or do you think they will go their own way?
- *What goal do I pursue?* The preferred action also depends on your ambition to solve, reduce or accept the problem. Do you only want to tackle the problem, for example, or do you also see opportunities to make a good impression?
- *Within what time limit do I want results?* The choice of your actions also depends on the time frame within which you want to realize something. Do you want to make a short-term promotion, for example, or are you prepared to aim for the long term?

The coping techniques *active addressing problems* and *approaching situations emotionally*are regarded as solution-oriented strategies, which in the long term offer the best chance of effectively reducing and avoiding negative stress.

- *Situatie emotioneel benaderen:* je aanvaardt de situatie met de bijbehorende emoties. Je uit deze gevoelens bijvoorbeeld via kunst, meditatie, humor, schrijven, sport, dans, ... en, als je daartoe de behoefte voelt, lucht je je hart bij een boezemvriend(in).

- *Active addressing problems:* you investigate how you can effectively tackle the problem. You anticipate what can happen and, if necessary, ask others for advice.
- *Approaching situations emotionally:* you accept the situation with the corresponding emotions. You express these feelings, for example through art, meditation, humor, writing, sports, dance, ... and, if you feel the need, you ask yourbest friend for advice.

EXPERIENCE BURNOUT
THE CAR METAPHOR

Congrats! You have passed the theoretical part of our driving course. The finish is close by. We continue with a practical driving test.

As you know:*the proof of the pudding is in the eating*. You can sit behind the wheel of a driving simulator for the practical driving test. "*Brrr, no stress, is not it?*" I am joking. As yourinstructor, I comfortably settle next to you. During the car ride I will embody your negative beliefs.

For the sake of completeness, I also tell you that this state-of-the-art driving simulator is capable of displaying your thoughts and bodily sensations while you are driving. "*That promises to be fun, is not it*!", I am chuckling.

External expectation	I count on you to follow the GPS and drive to Rome within the preset time of 15 hours. Good luck!
Negative belief	"15 hours is very tight!", I hear you thinking aloud.
Stress	You feel a slight tension in your shoulders.
Negative belief	I wishper in your ear: "*You may not fail, because otherwise everyone will find you weak.*"
Action	You press the accelerator firmly.
Incident	Ahead you see a hitchhiker waving
Negative belief	"*Sorry, but you can not afford to lose time*", I say authoritatively.
Action	You give some extra gas and ignore the look of the lifter in your rearview mirror.
Incident	A kilometer further we end up in a traffic jam.
Stress	The tension in your shoulders increases and you become restless.
Negative belief	Again I wishper in your ear: "*You may not fail, because otherwise everyone will find you weak.*"
Action	You notice that you only have 5 minutes and you start driving on the hard shoulder.
Consequences	Your ar stopped by wailing sirens from a police car. The following message appears on the screen of the simulator: GAME OVER.

It is understandable that you are displeased, but I know how to convince you not to let go of courage.

You try again a few times, but all your attempts fail. Each time the driving simulator comes up with a new obstacle: you lose time by refueling, you end up in the roadside due to a dangerous overtaking maneuver, you fly out of the corner by not keeping to the speed limit, ...

I softly lay my hand on your shoulder and say "*You are burdened with high expectations and negative beliefs (= in this example: I must not fail).*

But, believe me, there is a way out! Look inside and be open to other opinions." You answer hesitantly:"*I feel that my body is* **revolting***. It is not an unknown voice. I heard him before, but in the past I have silenced him.*"

Suddenly you take a groundbreaking decision. You ask me not to sit next to you during the following ride. "*Then I have at least no problems with your compelling, disturbing statements that I absolutely have to succeed in this assignment because otherwise people would find me weak!*",you say spontaneously.

Before you leave, you reveal to me, with the necessary justified pride, the new, positive beliefyou will use to convince yourself: "*Others may find me nice or annoying, but the quality of my life is only determined by how I think about myself !* "

"*Wow, that sounds promising!*", I react with admiration as I hopefully crawl out of the car.

External expectation	I count on you to follow the GPS and drive to Rome within the preset time of 15 hours. Good luck!
Positive belief	*"I can do it! There are many roads that lead to Rome!"*
Stress	You feel a positive tension because of the challenge.
Positive belief	*"Driving safely and pleasantly is more important than meeting the expectation of others to arrive in time!"*
Action	You drive further quietly.
Incident	Ahead you see a hitchhiker waving.
Positive belief	*"Driving safely and pleasantly is more important than meeting the expectation of others to arrive in time!"*
Positive belief	*"I would like some company during such a long trip!"*, you think aloud.
Action	You stop the car and invite the hitchhiker to ride along.
Stress	You feel cheerful because you are helping someone.

Incident	A kilometer further you will end up in a traffic jam.
Negative belief	Your old belief stands out again: "*I may not fail, because ...*"
Positive belief	"*It is normal that old beliefs do not surrender immediately. Just hold on and it will work!*"
Stress	You feel positive excitement and you are proud of yourself. You relax.
Incident	The hitchhiker is an Italian. He suggests a different route because it is more pleasant.
Positive belief	"*You think this is a good idea, because you have decided that the way of driving is more important to you than meeting the external expectation of following a certain route at a certain speed.*"
Action	You follow the advice of the hitchhiker and after 18 hours you arrive in Rome via a different road than the GPS had suggested.
Simulator	To your surprise, the driving simulator this time reports: MISSION SUCCEED.

"*How is it possible that I passed the driving test, although I am late and have not followed the route suggested by the GPS?*",you react surprised.

"*I must confess something!*", I reply with pubic cheeks. "*The driving simulator is designed so that the assignment is not feasible for anyone. The real intention is not to complete the task correctly. The only thing that matters is the score on the stress meter. If the simulator determines that you are safely in Rome, according to traffic regulations and without negative stress, then you have passed your driving test and have learned how to reduce stress and avoid a burnout by, for example, dealing critically with external expectations and by generating positive beliefs."*

By moving aside negative beliefs, such as "*failure is a sign of weakness*", positive beliefs, such as "*failure says nothing about who I am as a person*", can step out of their shadow.

If these new beliefs are helpful, the chronic negative stress decreases and the carpetisunrolled for effective emotions and effective actions. The risk of burnout decreases.

GO FOR SELF-REALIZATION

In the chapter '*Unmask the meaning of your life*'wehave already proposed self-realization as the main goal of your and everyone's existence.

Self-development, self-discovery, self-realization, ... all these concepts emphasize the importance of just being who you are, independent of the judgments and expectations of others and, perhaps even the most difficult of all, independent of self-criticism.

We opt for the term 'self-realization' to emphasize that your purpose in life is not limited to '*discovering who you are*', but must be extended to '*try out who you can become*'.

> *"Life isn't about finding yourself.*
> *Life is about creating yourself."*
> **- George Bernard Shaw -**

In *self-discovery* you see yourself as a lump of wood. You try to remove everything that does not belong to you so that your true self becomes visible.

In self-realization you behold yourself like a lump of clay. You have more opportunities than with a lump of wood to give your personality the shape you want. You decide who you want to become! The characteristics of clay, such as quantity, hardness, ... only impose insignificant limitations on your creativity and daring.

In the process of self-realization, the concept of 'self-confidence'
plays an important role. Here we opt for a definition in which we
describe self-confidence as 'growing in loyalty to yourself'.

You decide which of your talents you want to develop instead of
leaving these decisions to others or to external factors such as
the advertising world. In this way you also develop authenticity,
another important aspect of self-realization.

> *"A real personality is hard to recognize,*
> *because he does not look like anyone."*
> **- Cor de Jonghe -**

Self-realization as a life purpose should not be confused with
individualism. It is the intention to form a richer whole withall
people together. Through abundant connections between its
members, humanity as a whole can develop wider and deeper.

CALCULATE YOUR STRESSLEVEL

When we are ill, the thermometer tells us how serious it is, but unfortunately there is no stress meter that exactly indicates how much stress we have.

The Life Events Scale by Holmes and Rahe gives you an idea of your stress level. Holmes and Rahe have described radical events that can occur in a lifetime, in order of impact. The higher the score, the harder it is to deal with it in a healthy way and the greater the chance of negative stress, burnout or depression.

Life Event	Value	Life Event	Value
Death of a spouse	100	Foreclosure or mortgage or loan	30
Divorce	73	Change in responsibilities at work	29
Marital separation	65	Son or daughter leaving home	29
Jail term	63	Trouble with in-laws	29
Death of a close family member	63	Outstanding personal achievement	28
Personal injury or illness	53	Spouse begins or stops work	26
Marriage	50	Begin or end school	26
Fired at work	47	Change in living conditions	25
Marital reconciliation	45	Revision of personal habits	24
Retirement	45	Trouble with boss	23
Change in health of family member	44	Change in work hours or conditions	20
Pregnancy	40	Change in residence	20
Sex difficulties	39	Change in schools	20
Gain of new family member	39	Change in recreation	19
Business readjustment	39	Change in church activities	19
Change in financial state	38	Change in social activities	18
Death of a close friend	37	Mortgage or loan of less than $100,000	17
Change to a different line of work	36	Change in sleeping habits	16
Change in number of arguments with spouse	35	Change in number of family get-togethers	15
Home mortgage over $100,000	31	Change in eating habits	15

Even because of small, but always returning life events your stress bucket can overflow. It is therefore advisable to carefully plan important life decisions.

For example, after changing jobs, it is advisable to store your moving away plans.

It is also striking that events that are seen as fun and pleasant can also bring concerns. Just think of getting married, taking a vacation, family expansion and even Christmas.

How can you apply this scale to your concrete situation? Mark the events that occurred to you in the past year and add the number of points to determine your score. Recurring events alsocountthatnumber of times.

- More than 300 points: very much chance of stress.
- Between 150 and 300 points: much chance of stress.
- Less than 150 points: mild to moderate chance of stress.

If, for example, you lost a partner (= 100) during the past year and you became ill (= 63), you will have a great chance of experiencing stress.

As you now know, *activating events* are only instances and stress is determined by the way you judge situations, by your beliefs.

If, for example, you can give the loss of your partner a place in your life, because it came after a long, persistent illness, then there will only be slight or moderate stress.

Building these positive beliefs requires a lot of resilience and, moreover, a high acceptance capacity.

It is understandable and sometimes difficult to avoid that our life ship can capsize through a succession of storms and hurricanes.

UNDERSTAND HOW
BEHAVIOR WORKS

In the final room of *the comprehending phase* there are several exercise bikes. The exhibition on burnout aims to make its visitors aware of the fact that action is the key to putting the theory into practice. After all, we do not want to limit our actions tocircling thoughts in our head.

"If there is no action,
Then you have not made a real decision."
- Tony Robbins -

"Does it sound nice to cycle for half an hour?", I ask invitingly. You accept my offer and take place on a bicycle with a beautiful view of the garden. On your right side there is an empty seat for me.

"While we paddle quietly, I will explain to you the links between an activating event and behavior", I announce enthusiastically. *"But,"* you respond reprehensibly, *"that is multitasking!"* *"Yes, indeed,"* I reply with a satisfied grin, *"you are absolutely right. Multitasking is on the list of prohibited products. Hopefully you do not mind that I have put youto the test."*

After our bike ride, in silence of course, and a short break, I start my story about the factors that play a role in the development of behavior.

May I ask you to recall the cycling experience and to imagine which elements actually play a role during a bike trip. While

cycling the chain moves by pedaling, but also inside your body
a chain reaction occurs.

We go over the elements that are related to behavior.

- *Event*: something takes place. Events are changes in
  your environment. For example, you get a flat
  tirewhilecycling.
- *Sensations*: you become aware of something while
  cycling. Your senses (= hear, see, smell, taste and feel)
  perceive stimuli from your surroundings. You hear
  someone calling, you look at the sea, you smell the sea
  air, you taste and feel raindrops, ...
- *Thoughts and beliefs*: you realize or think of something.
  For example, you find that you are always unlucky.
- *Feelings*: you feel something. This is about emotions.
  Often different feelings are present at the same time. You
  are sad, angry, afraid, embarrassed or happy because
  you have a flat tire.
- *Behavior*: you do something. This includes everything
  you do. For example, you call for help, you shyly smile at
  a passerby, you throw your bike on the ground, ...
- *Consequences*: your behavior causes something. By
  your actions or by not taking any actions, you have an
  impact on situations and you can, in turn, cause or try to
  provoke new events. For example, someonecomesto
  your aid.

You can consider a *consequence* as a new event. So the circle
is complete and everything starts all over again.

"Fascinating! Very interesting, " younotice cleverly," but what does this knowledge help me with regard to the approach and prevention of stress and burnout? "

"*If your life runs smoothly, you rarely ask yourself which raw materials have contributed to this*", I answer convincingly. "But, if *your existence shows cracks, you will immediately look for cement or other ways to tackle the problem as good as possible.*"

Events, sensations, thoughts and beliefs, feelings, behaviors and consequences are the six building blocks with which you, as an architect, have to do the job of organizing your life in a valuable way.

Thoughts and beliefs can be windows so you can glance through familiar walls, allowing you to explore new horizons. They determine whether you will actually put a hand on the door handle with your behavior to step into another life.Thoughts and beliefs can also function as roller blinds, obstruct your view of new possibilities and lead to passivity or wrong actions.

Sensations and *feelings* act as a doorbell or as a knock on the window (*sometimes we even need an alarm = burnout*) to wake you up, so that you contact an architect to place extra windows (= *positive beliefs*) and to remove roller blinds (= *negative beliefs*).

COMMITMENT PHASE

DO NOT START TO SOON

There is no burnout meter to correctly determine when you can get back to work. Follow your instinct. Do not start working until you feel able to do so. Discuss this thoroughly with your family members, your doctor, the company doctor and your supervisor.

Dealing with stress will always remain a balancing act. You may be justifiably proud of your increased skills, but the risk of a burnout is always around the corner. Keep in mind that colleagues, friends and family members can not always assess what you can and can not handle. Be honest with yourself and others. You have nothing to prove. Clearly indicate your limits.

Realize that you have changed. **You have made a you turn**. That was also the intention of a burnout. You are now living with a different belief system. Your needs hierarchy has also undergone a thorough rearrangement. And your environment will need time to adapt to your new self.

After a burn-out the most important question regarding your work is: "*Do I still want that job?*" And if so: "*Am I sufficiently changed to be able to cope with that job or do I see possibilities to choose responsibi:ities that better suit me?*"

In second instance you have to check whether it is still possible to return. What is the position of your company regarding your return?

Try to start gradually (eg 25%) and build step by step to a level that is feasible and desirable for you.

In some cases, another job is the best option, but that is not always the case. Investigate what is essential and decisive for you and then evaluate realistically whether this is feasible. Try to gather information in advance to check whether the new company meets your needs.

It is useful to draw up a list of questions to determine whether a particular job is suitable for you. Answer each question with a rating (1 = necessary, 2 = very important and 3 = reasonably important).

The questions below may be eligible. Most of the points will already sound familiar to you in the meantime.

- Is the remuneration fair?
- Is there a pleasant working atmosphere?
- Is there sufficient attention for safety?
- Do you have room to put your own accents?
- Is there a threat due to restructuring, for example?
- Are there enough moments for rest and relaxation?
- Are you sufficiently appreciated for your efforts?
- Which values are central?
- How do social contacts go?
- …

CONVINCE YOURSELF
OF POSITIVE BELIEFS

<u>Origin of beliefs</u>

When we become aware of our perceptions, we speak of thoughts. We believe them to be true. Thoughts that are confirmed by events or by behavior grow in strength and change into *beliefs*. Just like behavior through repetition changes into automatic habits.

From beliefs we assume that they are correct, for example: "*I never expect to find a new job again, because all my attempts to date have failed.*" Experiences are an important breeding ground for the emergence of beliefs. They make a big mark on your reactions in the present, because you have a tendency to expect the same as what you have experienced before.

Having insight into the realization of beliefs and making them work to your advantage is the most important skill you need to avoid or reduce stress and burnout.

As you already know,your thoughts and beliefs determine how you experience an activating event.

When a loved one dies, you can think "*This can not and may not happen*". You can then get digestive complaints, feelings of sadness, the wish that it did not happen, the expectation that you will not easily get over this loss, so you will stay idle in your bed, ...

For example, if a death due to illness was expected, you can usually accept this more easily because you have other thoughts. Because of this, it is possible that you, despite the sadness, can continue to work and suffer less from painful physical complaints.

Also your expectations, opinions of others and the culture in which you live have a great influence on the formation of your beliefs.

Opinions can be so strong that you only perceive what you believe. What does not fit within your belief system is not perceived or transformed so that it corresponds with your beliefs. This way beliefs can be the maps of the past that predict and even determine your future.

Your impotency will become stronger if you declare yourself powerless by linking what is or is not possible to the past, circumstances, others or your own character and abilities.

Time for new beliefs

How can you weaken the power of negative beliefs and perhaps even replace them by positive beliefs?

First you have to accept that, like everyone else, you have various disturbing views. People are naturally inclined to think in terms of obstructions. We focus more on the negative than on the positive. We often ask ourselves *"What can go wrong?"*

This basic attitude should be placed within an evolutionary perspective. The prehistoric man was constantly exposed to danger. So he was super happy with brains that were always looking for possible dangers in his environment. Despite the enormous progress that our brains have made, they still exhibit this primitive trait. We are saddled with outdated software in our brain.

Beware! Do not dare to use this as an excuse! Think of it as a challenge to challenge your genetic limits. Become the programmer of your own brain cells.

Start working with your ideas. Do not look at them through the glasses of right or wrong, but check whether they are helpful.

Ask yourself the questions below

- Does this belief supports me to be who I want to be?
- Does this view helps me to achieve my dreams?
- Does this position gives me a good feeling about myself?

If the answer is three times yes, the belief has passed the test and you can use it.

The more you roll with a snowball, the bigger it gets. This also happens when the behavior cycle "event, sensations, thoughts and beliefs, feelings, behaviors and consequences" keeps repeating itself. In time, fixed patterns of beliefs, moods and habits that determine your life automatically arise. For example, if you find yourself insecure, you will often feel more insecure and behave accordingly.

In our brain this translates into increasing and stronger connections that are more easily accessible than others, just as a forest path becomes wider and easier to access if more walkers make use of it.

The nerve connections of views that are discussed less closely, such as "*I am proud of myself*", decrease and become less decisive for your life. Just like forest paths diminish and decrease in accessibility when they receive less visitors.

New points of view, such as "*I have a right to more time for myself*", have to hit hard and frequently on the table to be accepted by your brain. This is because prevailing opinions, such as "*I have to take care of my parents first*", do not give up their position of power without struggle. A small forest road does not immediately become wider, because you walk there on Sunday only.

Yet you should not despair. Change is always possible. At the level of the brain we speak about *neuroplasticity*. This is the ability your brain has to create new connections and weaken existing connections. Your way of thinking and your actions are the main actors in this changing process.

In the forest, your intention to walk followed by your walking behavior will determine the view of the paths. Wide roads will become less accessible if you don't use themanymore and narrow roads will become more accessible if you are more likely to treat them with your presence.

Thoughts and behavior often go hand in hand.

"If men define situations as real,
they become real in their consequences."
- William Thomas -

Thoughts and beliefs become stronger when they receive confirmation through behavior. For example, if I think I will fail and my attempt do not achieve the result I want, than I am even more convinced of my ignorance.

If established opinions are not confirmed by behavior, they want to maintain their power by giving themselves the benefit of the doubt. For example, if I think I will fail, but my attempt is successful, then I can continue to think that I can not do anything if I declare it to be a success by favorable circumstances instead of giving my abilities the honor they deserve.

Nerve connections only change when new viewpoints are supported by behavior several times. Actions can reprogram your ideas and thus your brain, but this is a difficult and a lengthy process. To persevere, to persevere and to keep persevering is the message!

The stiffness of your brain also has an important advantage. Your brain thus ensures stability by allowing adjustments to take place only if they are confirmed repeatedly. This steadfastness is a necessary characteristic in our rapidly changing society.

In addition to the rigidity of your brain, there is another danger: *the halo effect.*

Negative beliefs are like rotten apples that can infect the whole brain basket. For example, if I fear being fired, I can also have the idea of being worth nothing. I may have the idea that I will not find other work, I can assume that it is my own fault, ...

If you do not intervene in time, physical chain reactions may occur such as pressure on your chest, diarrhea, vomiting, ... and avalanches of negative feelings such as fear, anger, disillusion, etc.

MAKE TIME FOR EXTRA SKILLS

Congratulations, your tool kit is now filled with new insights and effective techniques to reduce negative stress, but there is still enough space for the interesting tools below to protect you even better.

We will discuss the following handy tools to become more resilient in life.

- Track guiltfeelings.
- Teach yourself the self-compassion course.
- Get acquainted with the influence of words.
- Ensure a balanced life.
- Discover the five happiness buckets.
- Consider a problem as a message.
- Detectyourauthenticself.
- Take responsibility.
- Dare to show your vulnerability.
- Look for new questions.

TRACK GUILT FEELINGS

It is important to properly distinguish the difference between regret and guilt. Guilt is a gnawing feeling that signals that you have intentionally done something wrong with the intention of hurting someone else. In case of regret, there is no malicious intent. If you check your own feelings, you will find that you often, wrongly, feel guilt instead of regret.

By becoming aware of the fact that you did not want to hit someone intentionally, it is easier to accept that you have done something wrong. Everyone sometimes makes a mistake. That does not detract from who you are as a person.

Use this insight to have compassion with yourself and to take the necessary next step towards forgiveness of yourself. With others you can not force forgiveness. You can only show that you are sorry. Accept that people need time to forgive and sometimes are unwilling to give forgiveness.

Remember that forgiving someone is not the same as overlooking or minimizing something. What do we mean by *giving forgiveness*? With forgiveness, you do not minimalize the pain you have felt, but you try to assume that the other person at that time did not sufficiently understand the influence of his actions or did not have enough insight and / or skills to act differently.

Thanks to forgiveness you also take care of yourself. When negative feelings like anger, revenge, ...appear in your life, they have a serious, unnecessary damper onyour happiness. Through (self) forgiveness these heavy emotions decrease in strength.

TEACH YOURSELF SELF-COMPASSION

We can learn a lot from others, but also from ourselves. Consider the way you treat yourself. How do you react if something does not work? Are you going to criticize yourself or do you show understanding for your shortcomings? This brings us to the concept of *self-compassion*, an important daily course to follow with yourself as teacher and as pupil.

Compassion means that you notice that someone is suffering. You are moved by this and feel warmth, caring and the need to support the other person.

> *"Increase your circle of compassion,*
> *so that the whole nature is covered by it."*
> **- Albert Einstein -**

Self-compassion means that you look at yourself with compassion if you have a hard time, if something does not work or if you do not like something about yourself. You say to yourself: *"I have a hard time with this! How can I take good care of myself? "*

If you want to build a house in which (self) compassion can live, acceptance of imperfection and vulnerability is a necessary foundation. Warmth, understanding, caring and kindness are the main support walls. Make sure that you do not stumble and end up in the basement of self-pity and overcompensation.

With *self-pity* you are going to magnify problems. You get isolated on your mountain full of pity, because you think you are the only one with a big setback. With self-compassion you zoom out and you see the bigger picture. You put things in perspective and you feel connected to others who, like you, sometimes also go through a valley.

In case of *overcompensation* you accept too little that hurdles belong to life. You try to make up for every setback by rewarding yourself. Empowering yourself is of course fantastic, but do it only because you find yourself valuable and not as a counterweight to trials. Overcompensation can lead to unhealthy behavior such as unhealthy food, extreme alcohol consumption, indiscriminate materialism, ...

Self-compassion is strongly related to mindfulness. Then you bring yourself into a judgment less state of consciousness, in which you view your own thoughts and feelings as they are, without suppressing or changing them. This observing attitude ensures that you are not absorbed by emotions and ideas.

GET ACQUAINTED WITH
THE INFLUENCE OF WORDS

It is very busy in the next room and I accept your proposal to enjoy a cup of coffee. The smell of coffee reminds me of a funny anecdote.

During one of my first tours I accompanied a somewhat older English lady. We met at the coffee machine at the entrance of the museum. She resolutely approached me and said: "*Are you Don?*" I did not realize she was referring to my name and answered convincingly: "*Yes, thank you, I have just finished my cup of coffee!*" She laughed warmly and replied: "*On no, I meant, is Don Key your name?*"

As you can see and certainly have experienced several times yourself, language can be very confusing. But despite that ambiguity, words are incredibly valuable. They are your main tool to show how you judge circumstances, feelings and actions and what your wishes are.

Through your senses you receive stimuli from the outside world and/or from your own inner environment. Your brain will then analyze and interpret this information.

These observations may never be labeled as the truth, but you should only consider them as your own truth. There are two important factors, *selection* and *subjectivity*, which cause that perceptions are not a copy of the complete reality.

At every event a whole group of labels are screaming to be chosen. Due to the large amount of stimuli and the observation limits of your senses, a large part of the stimuli is not observed. Experiences, expectations, wishes, possibilities of our senses, ... create, so to speak, a zoom lens, through which you register only a part of the reality.

If, for example, I lose my wallet, then words like *bad luck, attention grabber, stupid, sloth fox, ...* are getting out of my language suitcase. Even during the loss of my money bracket, I make a choice by selecting *loss* as a label. I might as well have chosen *robbery* or *distraction* as a label.

When I get promotion, terms such as *happiness, pride, merit, envy...* are impatient in my language suitcase to be unpacked.

In the case of colleagues, words such as a *show-off, money-wolf, dishonest*, ...may emerge.

Besides a zoom lens you also own personal filters. We all have our own language suitcase. Just as a dive in the water causes a lot of waves, every incident is experienced differently by everyone, so we each pick out our own labels.

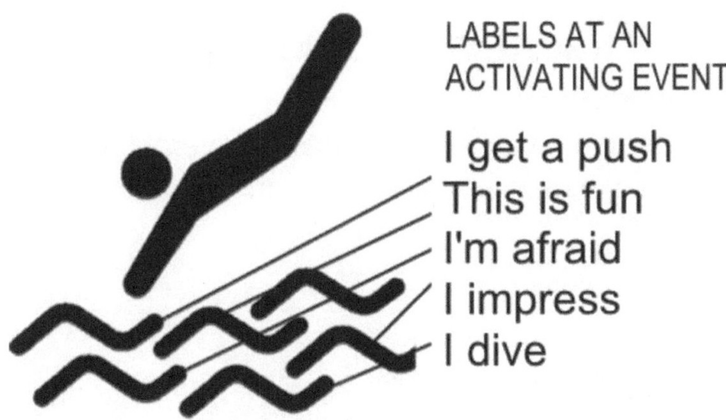

For example, you often have conflicts with your boss and therefore keep a close eye on him. You see him looking in your direction and you think you have done something wrong again. Your colleague rarely gets a comment and does not even notice that the boss is looking in her direction.

> *"Those who cannot change their minds*
> *cannot change anything."*
> **- George Bernard Shaw -**

The challenge we all face in the event of difficulties is to correctly assess which labels we use best.

In reality, *acceptance* and *resilience* often go hand in hand. For example, in order not to frustrate yourself unnecessarily, it is best to accept that arriving safely on time is not always feasible in the event of a flat tire. But you can also create resilient labels, such as: "*If I have a flat tire, I cannot always arrive on time, but I can inform you that I might be a little later.*"

ENSURE A BALANCED LIFE

When we enter the next room we receive several balloons. When we inflate them, we notice that eight balloons contain a specific word.

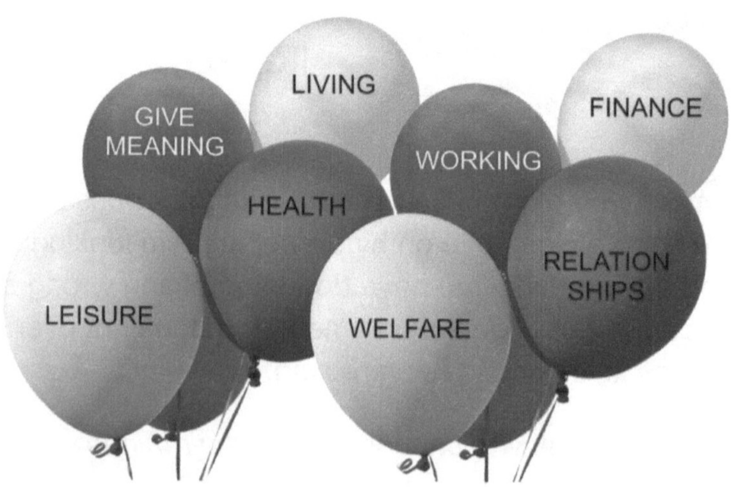

Give meaning, living, working, finances, leisure, health, welfare and relationships are essential areas of attention to regularly explore in your life.

If your life basket is only carried by one balloon, for example working, you are more vulnerable than someone who has several balloons to carry his life basket.

Here we end up with something fundamental. You cannot avoid that life sometimes brings unpleasant events on your path, but if you yourself take care of varied travel destinations, then your existence is more balanced. Then you can compensate one thing with an other. If, for example, you suddenly lose your job, you can receive support from your family, family and/or friends. Your free time can possibly act as an outlet.

If you neglect certain areas of life, for example your family or your health, or you spend too much time on one area of life, for example your work, you become entangled in it and it becomes increasingly difficult to change course.

DISCOVER THE FIVE HAPPINESS BUCKETS

Before the entrance of the next room, it is more a cabinet, a crowd waits patiently. It reminds me of the long queues in airports, where you have to hand over your suitcase.

"We will pay a visit to the happiness room", I reply in response to the question mark that appears on your forehead. This room is barely 1 square meter, so that people can experience that you do not need much to be happy. Every minute a bell sounds

and two new people can enter. The waiting time serves to make visitors aware of the fact that you do not automatically become happy. You have to make an effort to achieve it.

After waiting patiently - there are many fortune seekers after all - it is our turn. I give you some time to enjoy the masterpiece below that you can admire in the room of happiness and then I'll give you a brief explanation.

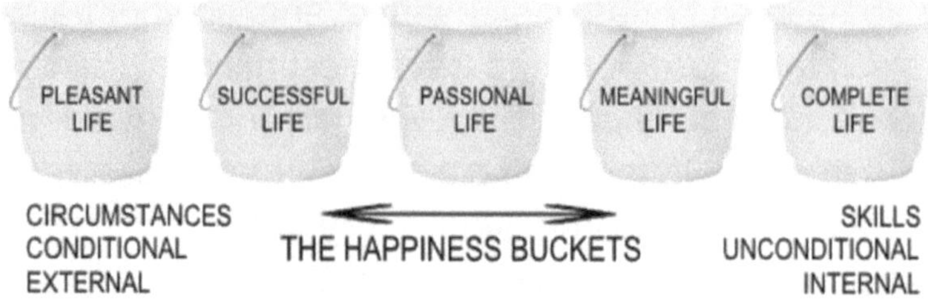

Happiness moves across a line between two extremes.

With *conditional happiness* you depend on *external circumstances* to feel happy. You then live as a sailor who can only experience well-being in favorable wind. Here happiness is highly result-oriented and absolute. You are happy or you are unhappy.

With *unconditional happiness, internal skills* determine how happy you feel. You then live as a sailor who experiences well-being by testing, by trial and error, which sailing techniques produce a favorable result. Happiness is here process-oriented and relative. If something does not work, you can still be partially happy by being proud of your efforts. You are more or less happy.

On the happiness line we distinguish *fiveforms of happiness* that are closely related to our basic needs. We present them as happiness buckets: *pleasure, success, passion, meaningfulness and completeness.*

In analogy with the *life areas*, the best way to increase your total happiness in life is placing the lucky buckets alternately under the lucky tap. One lucky bucket is not more valuable than another. You can only compensate for a shortage in one bucket by filling another. You should therefore pay attention to all buckets.

When a bucket is full, there is no point in letting flow the water from the lucky tap in that bucket, because superfluous happiness flows away. Let's take money for example. Sufficient money is useful, but more and more money will not increase your happiness proportionally.

> *"It is not how much we have,*
> *but how much we enjoy,*
> *that makes happiness."*
> *- **Charles Spurgeon** -*

The more happiness is unconditional, internal and based on skills, the deeper the experience, but also the more difficult it is to achieve it. That is why it is also advisable to focus your lucky arrows on all buckets.

On your path to more self-realization, you gradually learn where your personal limit lies with every bucket.

The bucket that receives the most attention varies from person to person and also from period to period. As a young adult, for example, you are more focused on success and as a pensioner you usually think more about meaningfulness and completeness.

It is also necessary to point out the danger of allowing others to determine what you need to be happy. Just think of the influence of the advertising industry.

I will discuss with you the five happiness buckets below. This way you can check with yourself if there is no bucket that threatens to overflow or to stayempty.

The lucky bucket that stands for a pleasant life

Singing along with a song on the radio, spontaneously grabbing your partner for a hug, making time for a nice chat, playing with the children, playing at cards with friends, ... are examples of small moments of happiness that have a big influence on yourgeneral well-being. The proverb *many little ones make a big* is an essential characteristic of happiness. You do not have to look for happiness in terms of big, bigger, biggest, ...

Pleasure activates your happiness hormone. It is the oil that makes your life engine laugh and shine. For people with a burnout, it is essential to provide themselves daily with these small happiness portions.

Joy helps to recharge the batteries, but cannot eliminate the problems. So make sure that you do not systematically look for fun to avoid difficulties.

The lucky bucket that symbolizes success

You can also derive happiness from success. You then experience satisfaction because of a social status based on things that you have realized. Then there is a feeling of appreciation, recognition and admiration.

This bucket is vulnerable. There can quickly arise a gap and the your success will flow away.

In order to fully enjoy this bucket, it is necessary to look at success in a special way.

Be proud of everything you have sown, the experiences you are richer and the moments of joy that you have experienced. Focus less on the fruits that your work has yielded. Too much striving for success as a goal creates a life with a lot of stress and fear of failure.

The lucky bucket that radiates passion

Passion arises if the external circumstances in which you find yourself correspond to the internal capacities that you have. At these moments you experience a mix of inspiration and control, also known as flow. Doing what you want to do and what you are good at, gives joy and positive energy. People are absorbed by their passion.

In passion, however, there is the danger of exaggeration, in which passion changes into obsession. It is also unrealistic to expect that everything in life can happen with passion

The lucky bucket that contains meaningfulness

Happiness comes about here through connectedness. Meaningfulness arises when you feel yourself an active and constructive part of a larger whole by transcending your individual interests and serving the general goal. This creates a positive feeling of deep connection, fulfillment and satisfaction. Realize that it is impossible to always experience the sense of meaningfulness.

The lucky bucket that strives for completeness

The deepest happiness experience embraces maximum sense of reality. The trick is to live completely in harmony with the reality that surrounds you. This is the result of a successful self-realization. Everything feels right as it is.

CONSIDER A PROBLEEM AS A MESSAGE

The next room is brightly lit. Fortunately, we have sunglasses on hand. Are you going on a trip to the sun or to the snow, sunglasses will come in handy. What is so special about sunglasses? When the sun shines, the strong sunlight will prevent you from seeing well. With sunglasses you do not change the strength of the sunlight, but you do not suffer from it anymore.

If you want to live a happy life, you also need such sunglasses. This is a basic attitude that ensures that you formulate obstacles in a different way. You will no longer label difficulties as problems, but as challenges you want to address.

A problem is not an enemy you want to disable, but someone with whom you want to engage in a conversation to find out why he speaks war language.

If you interpret the message in the right way and act accordingly, the emotional charge will change from disturbing to challenging and inviting.

Realize that you do not want a vacuum cleaner that sucks up all your problems, because that is an impossible fight. After all, difficulties are part of our lives.

Problems are asking for a new lifestyle in which you slow down, make more time for yourself and put into perspective the importance of some of your actions, such as earning a lot of money or gaining status.

For example, you can see anger and hatred as a deep need for respect or a need for recognition of your suffering.

Sadness for the loss of a loved one, for example, may indicate the need to mean something to someone, the need to connect with others or the desire for security now that reality makes you realize that your future will look different.

Fear, finally, can be labeled as a demand for more patience, because time brings advice. Fear can also be a need for support from others or a need for self-acceptance, in which your limitations are no longer afraid of daylight. Worrying can be seen as a need to do it right, as a need for security or as a hidden question of predictability

If you do not look for the message behind problems, obstacles will continue to present themselves. An obstacle hides a need that requires attention.

The primitive man did need problem-oriented thinking. With him everything revolved around survival. His sensations, thoughts, feelings, instincts, ... were always stand-by for one main assignment: "*Is there a problem? And if so, how do I solve it? For example, how can I satisfy my hunger? Where can I hide from the bad weather? What do I do when a wild animal approaches me?*" So the modern man still has that same reflex at manyevents:"*What can go wrong? And if so, how do I handle it?*"

We are champion in focusing on shortages: "*What is missing in my life? What do I want to achieve? Who do I want to become? What could be better?*"

Our consumer society is grateful for this attitude. The marketing boys and girls make usbelieve that we miss something important and they can give it to us at a very favorable price

If you go along with their story and think that you will be happier once this shortage is gone, then you are sufficiently brainwashed as a fortune seeker. You will wander around in all kinds of labyrinths of superfluous needs constructed by advertising, such as look young, own the latest mobile phone, wear designer clothing, ...

To live without shortages we often make great efforts and we are prepared to make high sacrifices. This gives us a backpack full of stress! We continuously live on the boundaries of our possibilities. If we compare our body with a car, the meter of the petrol tank is always in the red. We refuel every now and then, but continue to pressurize ourselves, making it difficult to get out of the red danger zone. The risk of feeling bad, for example due to depression or a burnout, hangs over our head like the Damocles sword. Living in the red zone costs tons of energy.

When a problem is resolved, we feel an overwhelming, intense sense of joy, euphoria, pleasure, lust, ecstasy, ...and we think that the bad feeling is gone forever. Soon this positive experience ebbs away and the unpleasant mood comes back. Realize that a disturbing feeling is never really gone. It was simply temporarily numb and pushed to the background.

DETECT YOUR AUTHENTIC SELF

I warn you when you enter the next room: "*Please note, this room is very confronting!*" You immediately understand what I mean. All walls are equipped with mirrors. It is impossible to escape yourself.

People are looking for their true identity from birth. The most frequently asked question is: "*Who am I?*" This question has a big disadvantage. There is a danger that you look at yourself in a too static way as if you could only be one person.

That is why I propose to look at yourself with the question: "*Who would I like to be?*" This offers many more possibilities. For example, it is important for parents to take care when raising their children that they do not impose their own values or popular societal tendencies.

The true building blocks of your identity are not your skills such as a good singing voice, but the values with which you want to connect yourself.

> "'Who am I'works paralyzing
> as a too small cage.
> 'Who do I want to be' gives me wings
> to explore the world."
> **- Don Key -**

I give you a few examples of values so that you can already feel a little bit where I want to go. Honesty, authenticity, respect, loyalty, creativity, admiration, commitment, love, gratitude, self-development, satisfaction, inspiring others, freedom, justice, ... are for many people guiding life values.

This list of values can continue indefinitely, but you are not a better person because your list is longer. Do not compare yourself with others in the field of value realization. Do not make your existence a match with winners and losers. Your life is not your opponent, but it is full of challenges that stimulate you to discover your unique potential in its completeness.

By looking for the oppressive sheaths in your life, such as what others expect from you, what society imposes on you, ... you can step by step reveal yourself and search for the butterfly in yourself, which is unique and perfect is.

It is therefore essential to clearly see the difference between *equality* and *equivalency*.

We are all a different puzzle piece of the big puzzle called humanity. We are therefore not equal and that is not the intention either. Realize that there are no beautiful or ugly puzzle pieces. There can only be missing or unnecessary puzzle pieces if you try to be someone else than yourself.

Our society threatens to become a puzzle with too many duplicate puzzle pieces such as luxury, status, appearance, ... but also with numerous missing links such as love, tolerance, honesty, goodness, satisfaction, ...

If you cultivate your individuality, you make yourself richer, but also society as a whole. Self-realization is the overarching goal of life for everyone!

It is strange that we often put people on a scale and make comparisons with labels such as the best, the fastest, the most beautiful, the coolest, the sweetest, the smartest, ... We are even placed under the microscope before birth and compared to others and with statistical standards such as *"He will be as big as his father", "She will hopefully become a better swimmer than me, ..."*

As a result, differences are labeled as unequal. You will then receive winners and losers. A preferential treatment arises whereby certain characteristics become the norm and get a stage and other characteristics are denied the opportunity to show themselves. This makes it difficult for values at the bottom of the ladder to climb up.

By encouraging certain qualities, for example intelligence, and not supporting other qualities, for example creativity, you get a narrow society that cannot respond adequately to changes.

Comparing yourself with someone else is no problem if it serves to admire that person for his uniqueness. As long as you do not feel the urge to become that other person or to be better, there is nothing wrong with making comparisons.

Due to the great diversity between people, complete self-realization is not feasible. If you also want to take account of others, you sometimes have to give up a piece of your individuality. The challenge of our society is to ensure that we all have equal opportunities to develop our uniqueness. Characteristics such as acceptance, for example "*I cannot shout everywhere*", and tolerance, for example "*I understand that children sometimes make noise*", are necessary in order to give each member of our society equal opportunities to grow.

Give people freedom, within a negotiable space, and teach them that that freedom brings responsibility. This means that there are consequences associated with violating agreements. After all, there will always be a limit (necessary) within which you can and must shape your uniqueness.

Moreover, mankind, as ruler of the planet earth, also has the task of offering equal opportunities to systems like the animals, plants, environment, and so on. The thorough disruption of one important system can endanger the survival of our planet.

When you connect with your authentic role, life suddenly runs smoother. You then come more and more into the flow of your existence, because you no longer try to imitate others.

When you walk away from your identity, to belong to a group, you become a stranger in your own life. It is logical that this will never lead to satisfaction. By connecting yourself, via friendship or love, with others, you open doors to enjoy each other's authenticity.

How can you shamelessly be completely yourself? How can you convincingly say to your mirror: "*I am good enough!*"

As you know, things, people and activating events have no meaning, but they become relevant through the labels we give them. If someone likes me for example, then that is not a fact, but an opinion. I cannot be smart, beautiful, just or helpful. I can only link those qualities to myself or others can think that those characteristics belong to me.

Realize that this labeling system is your most important tool for feeling valuable. You decide completely which values you assign to yourself, but also which labels you accept from others and which you do not accept. *You are or becomethe person you choose to be!*

The feeling "*not being good enough*" arises in your childhood. As a child your thinking ability is still insufficiently developed. You think black and white. Something is correct or something is wrong. It is true or false. Moreover, as a child you do not make a distinction between '*what you do*' and '*who you are*'. You make generalizations. You don't put things in perspective. Behavior thus gets the stamp of a character trait!

This process is sometimes encouraged by others, such as parents, teachers, friends, ...If you do something wrong, you can get the message to be stupid instead of just doing something wrong. For example, if you have not cleaned up your toys, you are a sloth instead of your behavior being criticized as laziness. If you do not wear designer clothes, for example, you are a loser instead of someone who prefers other clothes. Although we also get positive reactions, a feeling of "*I'm not good enough*" grows with everyone, to a greater or lesser extent.

What happens now if you pronounce the sentence "*I am not good enough*"? You then make a comparison between yourself and certain norms that live in society and in groups with whom you come into contact and where you want to be part of. Moreover, you erroneously assume that these standards are the only correct ones and that you are obliged to follow them.

Disconnect yourself from the opinions of others. Their views only say how they experience you. With their ideas about you they only tell something about themselves and nothing about you. Learn to look at yourself in a different way. No longer see yourself as a sum of present and missing qualities and opinions of others, but as a person who has committed himself to fundamental values such as creativity, patience, tolerance, ...

TAKE RESPONSIBILITY

At the entrance of the next room hangs a sign with the message: "*Enter on your own responsibility!*" You enter firmly and shoutsurprised: "*This room is empty! That does not make any sense?*"

I answer your question with a counter question: "*How do you win the lottery?*" After a short reflection time, you hesitantly come up with the following answer: "*If I'm lucky and the numbers on the balls match those on my lottery form.*"

That is true, but do not forget that first of all you have to fill in a lottery form. Without actions you are completely dependent on circumstances in life. Only by taking responsibility and taking a certain action - for example entering a room or filling out a lotto form - something can change in your favor.

Activating events - such as an unexpected delay - put your life on certain railways, but each individual decides for himself whether he is a passenger and undergoes the situation or becomes a machinist andchoose a different path through his own way of thinking

You are responsible for the meanings you give to the situations in your life. A delay can be a stumbling block, something that destroys a trip, or a challenge or something that offers opportunities such as extra time to check a number of things?

Some chances fall from the sky, but mostly you have to create them yourself!

"If opportunity doesn't knock,
build a door."
- Milton Berle-

<u>**Growing towards more responsibility**</u>

Even a baby does not escape responsibility. Just think of a baby who cries when he is hungry. Of course, parents care most during this phase of life. With an ideal upbringing, the child is guided step by step in taking responsibility.

From a legal point of view, in most countries, you are considered as adult from the age of eighteen. You will then be labeled as fully responsible for all your actions, except of course for people with mental disabilities.

You need that responsibility to achieve a certain degree of independence, creating room for your own happiness path. The life ball is in your camp. If you want change in your life, you have to take the initiative yourself. Of course - and there is nothing wrong with that - you can ask others or society to help you with this. You also sometimes have to put aside certain characteristics - for example misplaced pride - and accept help from others.

There are thousands of legal texts that determine who is responsablein a certain situation, but we do not go into that subject. It is, however, interesting to emphasize that extra opportunities often arise if you turn the rudder yourself instead of waiting for a favorable wind.

If you feel that your responsibility is being restricted too much by well-intentioned parents, family members, colleagues and/or friends, it is your job to point this out.

You best deal with this difficult task by first thanking them for being concerned about you.Then you ask them for understanding. You try to make it clear to them that you choose to determine the direction of your life yourself. Unfortunately, it is not always possible to achieve this without a conflict.

A problem that many people encounter, after a major event, is that they shift responsibility to others or to society.

Postponement is also such a pitfall. If you postpone something, be critical of yourself. Do not put your head in the sand. Many situations worsen when people flee responsibilities. Combine this with gentleness and do not condemn yourself.

> *"I placed my scale in the corner*
> *and told him he could only come out*
> *if he would apologize."*
> ***- Author unknown -***

DARE TO SHOW YOUR VULNERABILITY

Suddenly my cell phone comes to life. Ideally I would just leave my mobile at home, but there are family members and friends with whom I have a strong bond and with whom I want to stay connected. Fortunately, I can decide autonomously with each call whether I want to commit or not.

In daily life you stand - almost continuously - for the choice: *to connect or not to connect!* You maintain relationships with other people, but do not forget your contacts with animals, nature, society and of course yourself. How about the love you give to your partner, the friendship you get from your dog, the support you receive from your best friend, the attention you give to your garden, the courage you give yourself in case of difficulties.

Imagine we represent *connecting* as puzzling. You start puzzling full of expectations, but you soon notice that it does not always click. Sometimes you find a puzzle piece that fits, sometimes it does not work and it can also happen that you have doubts.

Also in real life there are no guarantees in the field of connections. Relationships can enrich your life, but you can also make bad connections or something in between.

We all realize that connections make an important contribution to our happiness in life. It is less clear to know what we really need to achieve profound relationships that substantially enrich our lives. We therefore take a moment to consider the concepts of *vulnerability* and *equivalency*.

Real connections and vulnerability

A knight uses a harness to protect his vulnerability. In relationships you can try to achieve this by denying, hiding or minimizing your limitations or your otherness.

Defraying, masking or weakening your vulnerability is an understandable reaction, but also a two-edged sword. For example, you can protect yourself from grief or disappointment by closing yourself from others, but then you also deny yourself experiences as deep joy or intense understanding.

Vulnerability is like opening your front door after someone has rung. Because of the size of the door opening you control your vulnerability in relation to the person who rings the bell. For example, if you leave the door ajar, the other person can hurt you less, but there is, for example, insufficient room for an embrace. It is understandable and also justifiable that in new contacts you first adopt a cautious attitude and increase the door opening step by step as the trust within the relationship grows.

To obtain deep connections, mutual courage and willingness to show vulnerability will be needed. Only from openness something new and valuable can grow.

Connections and vulnerability are put to the test by criticism on your personality. There is a danger that people will dare to become less vulnerable because of this, making the relationship in question more superficial.

As you already know, your cannot control the reactions of others, but you can protect yourself against their negative influence by the way you interpret their reactions.

Assume the following view: "*Only I determine who I am. Others can at most indicate how they experience my behavior.*"People's opinions therefore only indicate whether or not you meet their expectations. If for example someone says: "*I find you slow!*", than he only says that he finds your pace slow compared to his expectations. Do not interpret that statement as a personal shortcoming. It is only your job to meet the wishes of others if you have made that choice yourself.

<u>**Real connections and equivalency**</u>

By promoting tolerance in the field of differences, education can help people to live more authentically. Shame, the fear of being rejected because you are not good enough, then disappears like snow in the sun. Get rid of that measurement society! Giving differences an equalvalue is one of the main challenges of each individual.

If you want to avoid pain or grief in a connection, then only superficial connections are feasible. The more your door is ajar, the more difficult contacts will be. Deep connections require more vulnerability, sometimes even a door that is wide open.

What is useful in terms of self-protection, is to check whether your vulnerability is in accordance with the type of connection you want. If you want an in-depth connection, limited vulnerability will make this impossible. If you are only looking for a superficial connection, do not open your door more than necessary.

Being vulnerable, can also be misunderstood, namely as a demand for a deeper connection. Be aware of this. Make sure you only ask the kind of connection you want.

During each connection there is a mutual harmonization of vulnerability. We scan each other's longings. Indicate clearly what you wish to receive and what you do not like. Give the other the space to freely determine what his needs are and what he is willing to invest. If the parties involved are insufficiently aware of this reconciliation process, you will get wrong expectations and disappointments that could have been avoided.

LOOK FOR NEW QUESTIONS

We end up in a room that is decorated as a fish pond. "*What is the purpose of this?*",you laugh surprised. "*Oh, this is a special fish pond*", I answer with a wink.

In life we often fish for answers to all kinds of questions, such as "*Why should this happen to me?*", but we rarely ask ourselves if our questions are meaningful. That's why we will not go angling for answers to all sorts of questions about life, but together we will try to catch interesting questions.

"Successful people have better questions
and as a result they get better answers."
- Tony Robbins -

"There is more wisdom in a new question
than in 1000 known answers."
- Don Key -

Repeatedly we ask ourselves circle questions, such as "*Why do I always have bad luck?*", so that we keep thinking in circles. We then end up on a path that we walk again and again. That road eventually changes into a swamp, in which we sink deeper and deeper.

It is important to analyze questions in advance. Do not immediately look for an answer when a question pops up in your head. First think about this question and consider: "*Can this question give me an answer that is helpful for me?*"

After this investigation it will often turn out that many questions lead to nothing. Consider such questions as small fishes and throw them back into the pond.

In addition, there are questions that only give your the options *yes or no*. These questions are similar to fishes that are too small to keep and too big to throw back. Whatever you do, you always feel that you are making a wrong choice.

Which questions are we looking for? Below you will find a number of examples of interesting questions. Since the intention is to answer them yourself, I have already mold them in the I-form for convenience.

To measure change, you can use *scale questions*. You then try to form a measurable picture of the severity of your problem. "*How annoying do I experience my current situation on a scale of 0 (not bad) to 10 (very bad)?*" This allows you to determine progress, stagnant or deterioration.

In addition to a scale question, it is useful to gauge your power sources. By doing so, you negate the thought - which you may have - that you are completely overwhelmed by your problem and completely powerless. A grateful power source question is: "What helps me to keep up?"

In addition, look for *exceptions*. No matter how seriously you experience your problem, there are always times when things go slightly uphill. Then consider the following: "*What other things am I doing at times when I feel a little better?*"

Regularly examine *your skills*. Just like this is the case with everyone, your life also has ups and downs. Go back in time and be aware of the following question again: "*What successful actions have I taken in the past in periods where I had difficulties?*"

Pay attention to *the smallest positive step*: "*What is - despite the difficult situation in which I find myself - already possible to make life more tolerable for me, without expecting that this will solve everything?*"

Imagine *the wonder question*. When exploring that wonder question, it is crucial that you only think about what you want and not about what you think is feasible. "*What do I see myself doing when the problem is solved? What do I want instead of my current difficulties?*"

Congrats! Now you have different meaningful questions hanging on your fishing hook. The cook in you can now get started to prepare various answers to these questions.

In summary, it is best to start from the following starting points.

- Consider achieved successes and not misses from the past. Do more of what works well or better. Put the focus on thedesiredsituation.
- Look for exceptions. When does the problem not occur or less, and what do you do differently at that moment or in that situation?
- Investigate your qualities to solve problems. How did you deal with such or similar problems in the past? Also look at what you do to stay upright in similar contexts.
- Work step by step. Small steps initiate a positive movement in the direction of the solution.

MAKE A CONTRIBUTION
AS AN EMPLOYER

Preventing unhealthy stress and burnouts is a shared responsibility of employees, employers, the government and the society.

Here we would like to draw attention to the tools that employers have at their disposal to reduce the chance of unhealthy stress and burnout among their employees.

Since 1 September 2014 every employer has the legal obligation to take preventive measures to reduce the risk of burnout.

As a boss you need to avoid the changing of your company into a COBRA-snake with Complexity,Overruling personality, Banishing stability, Risk taking and Ambiguity as main characteristics?

What are the key concerns for any business owner to create a healthy working environment?

Provide fewer incentives. You reduce the stress level by limiting stimuli, by not expecting people to be available all the time and by banishing multitasking.

Show appreciation and give constructive feedback. People are not machines. As an employer, make sure that your employees feel useful and are proud of their jobs. Provide them with a fair reward for their performance.

Provide a clear job description and task variation. It is crucial that employees know well what is and what is not expected of them. This increases their sense of security. Uncertainty quickly gives rise to a negative spiral, as a result one certainty is becoming stronger: the idea that uncertainties are increasing. Clarity translates into building blocks such as predictability, stability and simplicity.

An employer must *communicate clearly*, so that everyone knows why one employee, for example, gets a pay raise and the other does not. People are very sensitive to justice. Provide a fair evaluation system.

Provide sufficient autonomy. Employees experience much more job satisfaction and feel more fully treated when they have more freedom in the way they can fill in their work. Give them co-determination for important aspects such as the regulation of their working hours. It is also important that they do not have to account for everything. Give your staff confidence! People deal with stress better when they feel that they can shape their own values.

Pay plenty of attention to creating a collegial atmosphere where employees support each other. Teamwork is becoming increasingly important.

Finally, as an employer you may not lose sight of the work-life balance of your staff. This can be achieved, for example, by flexibility in working hours, both in terms of the number of hours and their spread.

CONSOLIDATING PHASE

STAND STILL AND LOOK AT THE FUTURE

We are on the highest floor: *the consolidating phase*. You've got your life back on track. You may follow a different track or at least your driving style has changed drastically. You have made the necessary U-turn. Yet the rest of your life remains - for a large part - a closed book.

Due to this lack of full transparency, a wrong choice is made quickly. This does not have to be a natural disaster, as long as you realize it is just a diversion. Therefore it is advisable not to dismantle professional support too quickly. It is clear that you want to avoid a second burnout at all costs.

Your future is what you deserve! And now you have learned that you largely determine that yourself. You bear the ultimate responsibility for your process of self-realization. You decide who you want to be. Conditions have only an influence on the duration and the level of difficulty of that process.

GO FOR IT

I hope you have had an instructive tour in our museum. For me personally it was a great satisfaction to guide you through this exhibition.

One last tip as a farewell present: "*Take enough time to understand everything. Reread some chaptersif necessary and then cautiously get to work with a number of ideas.*"

"The best way to predict your future
is to create it in the present."
- based on Abraham Lincoln -

Do not worry! You are sufficiently armed to protect yourself against burnout. You know which misleading paths you have to avoid and how you can build new ones.

Good luck and believe in yourself and maybe our paths will cross again in the future!

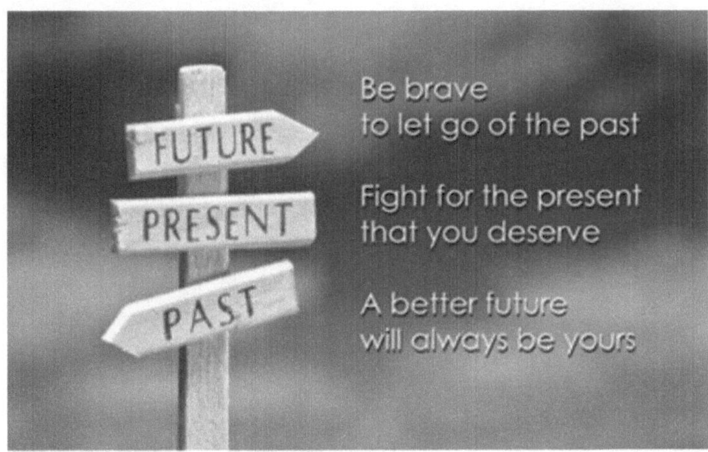

END OF EXHIBITION

LITERATURE LIST

Books

Dewulf Luk, Vangronsveld Guido – *Stop burn-out: wat als je batterijen leeglopen: praktische tips en technieken om burn-out te herkennen, te vermijden, te bestrijden*, Lannoo Campus, 2016.

Geraerts Elke –*Mentaal kapitaal: versterk je mentale veerkracht en vermijd burn-out*,Lannoo, 2015.

Hermans Henk –*Handboek Rationeel Emotieve Therapie*,Boom, 2011.

Lannoey Mieke –*Burn-out: het begin van verandering*, Ankhhermes, 2016.

Roelands Anita –*Nooit meer burn-out! In drie stappen leren genieten van werk en leven*, Uitgeverij S.W.P. B.V., 2017.

Swinnen Luc – *Burn-out: Boordevol tips om (opnieuw) plezier te beleven aan je werk*, Wpg Be Davidsfonds, 2012.

Swinnen Luc, Dirk Coeckelbergh–*1001 antwoorden op stress en burn-out*,Van Halewyck, 2017.

Verhulst Jan –*RET-jezelf: verstandig omgaan met problemen*, Pearson Benelux B.V., 2009.

Websites

www.confront.nl
www.kwadraet.be
www.onyourmind.nl
www.wereldmarketeers.nl
www.zelfcompassie.nl

www.ingramcontent.com/pod-product-compliance
Lightning Source LLC
Chambersburg PA
CBHW051449250726
48655CB00001B/319